GETTING YOUR LIFE BACK FROM NEUROPATHY

How to Restore and Regain Nerve Health

JOHN ZILLIOX DC.

Important Information for the Reader

This information presented in this book has been compiled from my clinical experience and research. It is offered as a view of the relationship between diet, exercise, emotions, and health. This book is not intended for, self diagnosis or treatment of disease, nor is it a substitute for the advice and care of a licensed health care provider. Sharing of the information in this book with the attending physician is highly desirable.

This book is intended solely to help you make better judgements concerning your long-term health goals. If you are experiencing health problems, you should consult a qualified physician immediately. Remember early examination and detection are important to successful treatment of all diseases.

TABLE OF CONTENTS

Chapter 1

WHERE UNITED STATES RANKS
IN QUALITY OF HEALTH CARE

U ntil the early 1990s, despite the accomplishments of certain high-income countries in achieving significant continued improvements in life expectancy at birth, there was considerable disagreement among gerontologists and demographers as to what the future might bring. On the one hand, pessimists believed that the deaths above age 80 were due to problems associated with senescence and intractable aging processes. Consequently, increases in longevity beyond age 85 or so were unlikely to be achievable without fundamental biomedical breakthroughs that would affect those processes themselves. On the other hand, optimists believed that continued improvements in life expectancy were to be expected and that the official population projections of the time were too conservative.

A lack of reliable and internationally comparable data initially limited demographers' ability to study patterns of mortality and morbidity at advanced ages. In the United States, for example, demographers have long been wary of using mortality data at older generations because of concerns about the quality of the data and the validity of age reporting.

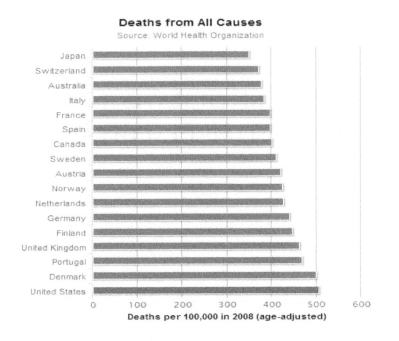

Deaths from All Causes
Source: World Health Organization

We've known for years that Americans tend to be overweight and sedentary and that our health care system, despite being the most expensive in the world, produces some less-than-plum results. Health nerds who closely follow the news may even have known that we live shorter lives than people in other wealthy nations and that infants in the U.S. die from various causes at far higher rates.

The report was prepared by a panel of doctors, epidemiologists, demographers, and other researchers charged by the National Research Council and the Institute of Medicine to better understand Americans' comparative health. They examined when and why people die in the U.S. and 16 other countries, including Australia, Japan, Canada, and nations in Western Europe. The data they pulled -- from such bodies as the World Health Organization and the Organization for Economic Cooperation and Development -- already existed, but no one had yet examined it this comprehensively.

The results surprised even the researchers. To their alarm, they said, they found a "strikingly consistent and pervasive" pattern of poorer health at all stages of life, from infancy to childhood to adolescence to young adulthood to middle and old age. Compared to people in other developed nations, Americans die far more often from injuries and homicides. We suffer more deaths from alcohol and other drugs and endure some of the worst rates of heart disease, lung disease, obesity, and diabetes.

These disproportionate deaths, primarily affect young people. For three decades, Americans, particularly men, have had either the lowest or near the lowest likelihood of surviving to age 50. The most powerful reasons found for that were a homicide, car accidents, other kinds of accidents, non-communicable diseases, and perinatal problems like low birth weight and premature birth, which contribute to high infant mortality.

Among the most striking of the report's findings are that among the countries studied, the U.S. has:

- The highest rate of death by violence, by a stunning margin
- The highest rate of death by car accident, also dramatically so
- The highest chance that a child will die before age 5
- The second-highest rate of death by coronary heart disease
- The second-highest rate of death by lung disease
- The highest teen pregnancy rate
- The highest rate of women dying due to complications of pregnancy and childbirth

The report does reveal bright spots: Americans are more likely to survive cancer or stroke, and if we live to age 75 we're likely to keep on living longer than others. But these advances are dwarfed by the grave shortcomings.

Where Does U.S. Rank In Crisis Care Intervention?

The World Health Report 2000, Health Systems: Improving Performance, ranked the U.S. health care system 37th in the world— a result that has frequently been discussed during the current debate on U.S. health care reform.

Despite having the most expensive health care system, the United States ranks last overall among 11 industrialized countries on measures of health system quality, efficiency, access to care, equity, and healthy lives, according to a new Commonwealth Fund report. The other countries included in the study were Australia, Canada, France, Germany, the Netherlands, New Zealand, Norway, Sweden Switzerland, and the United Kingdom. While there is room for improvement in every country, the U.S. stands out for having the highest costs and lowest performance—the U.S. spent $8,508 per person on health care in 2011, compared with $3,406 in the United Kingdom, which ranked first overall.

Despite the claim by many in the U.S. health policy community that international comparison is not useful because of the uniqueness of the United States, the rankings have figured prominently in many areas. It is hard to ignore that in 2006, the United States was number 1 in terms of health care spending per capita but ranked 39th for infant mortality, 43rd for adult female mortality, 42nd for adult male mortality, and 36th for life expectancy. These facts have fueled a question now being discussed in academic circles, as well as by government and the public: Why do we spend so much to get so little?

The current proposals for U.S. health care reform focus mostly on extending insurance coverage, decreasing the growth of costs through improved efficiency, and expanding prevention and wellness programs. The policy debate has been overwhelmingly centered on the first two of these elements. Achieving universal insurance coverage in the United States would protect households against undue financial burdens at the same time that it was saving an estimated 18,000 to 44,000 lives. However, narrowing the gap in health outcomes between the United States and other high-income countries or even slowing its descent in the rankings would require much more than insurance expansion.

Why Does Western Medicine Insist On Using Crisis Care Tactics For Prevention Situations?

Now that health care reform has been put on the back burner, maybe it is time to discuss what health care reform should look like. Although we talk about a "health care" system and health care reform, what we're actually talking about is a "disease care" system and disease care reform. Doctors of modern western medicine are trained to treat disease with drugs and surgery. They are not trained to keep people healthy.

At medical school, the doctors are taught how to treat the symptoms of the disease, rather than how to prevent disease in the first place. For example, throughout the training, they receive very few lectures on nutrition, despite the fact that diet is fundamental to good health. Nor are they trained in other lifestyle modalities that help keep people well, such as exercise and relaxation therapies. They are taught nothing about the wisdom of alternative medical systems that have been helping other cultures for centuries.

I will be the first to acknowledge that modern western medicine and science have made phenomenal advances. These improvements alleviate pain and suffering and save lives every day. Better treatment of trauma and burns for example, or the management of acute medical and surgical emergencies, are among the miracles of modern life. We have drugs today that, when used appropriately, work wonders. We are indeed blessed to have modern western medicine in our arsenal, and for disasters like the Haiti earthquake, this kind of medicine is life-saving.

In a true health care system, we must use modern western medicine for what it is good at - crisis care, acute medical and surgical emergencies - and natural, non-toxic and non-invasive therapies whenever possible. The most effective ways of preventing and treating most chronic diseases are diet, supplements, exercise, stress management and other benign modalities. And herein lies the rub. Although guidance may be helpful, lifestyle changes can't be imposed from above - they have to come from you. There is no greater reward than being the master of your health.

What Is The Origin Of Big Pharma? (When Did They Take Over)?

The term Big Pharma is used to refer collectively to the global pharmaceutical industry. According to Steve Novella, the term has come to connote a demonized form of the pharmaceutical industry. Professor of writing Robert Blaskiewicz has written that conspiracy theorists use the term Big Pharma as "shorthand for an abstract entity comprising corporations, regulators, NGOs, politicians, and often physicians, all with a finger in the trillion-dollar prescription pharmaceutical pie."

The Big Pharma conspiracy theory has four classic traits: first, the assumption that a small malevolent cadre perpetrates the conspiracy. Secondly, believe that the public at large is ignorant of the truth; thirdly, that its believers treat lack of evidence as evidence; and finally, that the arguments deployed in support of the theory are irrational, misconceived or otherwise mistaken.

Big Pharma is the pejorative nickname given to the pharmaceutical industry. Critics of the industry often use this nickname when discussing abuses by the industry, including:

- Trying to suck every penny out of the pockets of the sick, injured, dying, and hypochondriacs; Inventing new maladies so people will buy more drugs (as opposed to inventing better drugs so more people would become addicts);
- Censoring alternative treatments that would be cheaper or more effective, rather than patenting and industrializing them (much as proponents of free energy claim censorship by energy companies, without basis);
- Renaming old maladies, so people will think their conditions are more serious, making them more willing to pay higher prices for prescriptions.

There are scientifically-literate criticisms of Big Pharma. However, the overwhelming majority of criticism comes from non-scientific bases. Many alternative medicine merchants (such as homeopaths and naturopaths) stridently blame most or all opposition on Big Pharma, rather than, say, a lack of scientific evidence for their claims.

When Did Insurance Companies Come About?

The history of insurance consisted of the development of the modern business of insurance against risks, especially regarding cargo, property, death, automobile accidents, and medical treatment. The industry helps to eliminate risks (as when fire insurance companies demand the implementation of safe practices and the installation of hydrants), spreads risks from the individual to the broader community, and provides an important source of long-term finance for both the public and private sectors. The insurance industry is profitable and provides attractive employment opportunities for white-collar workers.

In the United States, health insurance is any program that helps pay for medical expenses, whether through privately purchased insurance, social insurance or a social welfare program funded by the government. Synonyms for this usage include "health coverage," "health care coverage" and "health benefits." In a more technical sense, the term is used to describe any form of insurance that protects against the costs of medical services. This usage includes private insurance and social insurance programs, such as Medicare, which pools resources and spreads the financial risk associated with major medical expenses across the entire population to protect everyone, as well as social welfare programs such as Medicaid and the Children's Health Insurance Program. Which assist people who cannot afford health coverage.

In addition to medical expense insurance, "health insurance" may also refer to insurance covering disability or long-term nursing or custodial care needs. Different health insurance provides different levels of financial protection, and the scope of coverage can vary widely, with more than 40 percent of insured individuals reporting that their plans do not adequately meet their needs as of 2007.

The share of Americans without health insurance has been cut in half since 2013. Many of the reforms instituted by the Affordable Care Act of 2010 were designed to extend health care coverage to those without it; however, high-cost growth continues unabated. National health expenditures are projected to grow 4.7% per person per year from 2016–2025. Public healthcare spending was 29% of federal mandated spending in 1990, 35% in 2000, and is projected to be roughly half in 2025.

Today, the internet has changed the insurance industry by blowing the field wide open. Now people can go online to find the cheapest rate, even as companies shop internationally for the right coverage. This is one source of motivation for companies to merge with other financial services. The increase in size gives them a global market and the integration of services gives them a domestic advantage with customers who are more concerned with convenience than price.

When Did Medical Doctors Go From Private Practices And Into Hospital Groups?

There is a dangerous trend underway in American healthcare: The death of the private practice doctor's office. This is a deliberate trend driven primarily by federal policymakers, and it does not bode well for either the cost of healthcare or the health of individual patients.

Hospitals justified their mergers by claiming they helped reach economies of scale. But the mergers also reduced competition, helping the hospital systems negotiate higher reimbursements from health insurers.Then came the A.C.A., which envisioned large, integrated provider networks, and the government was willing to hand out billions of dollars to providers that successfully implemented the government's vision of quality care.The effects on physicians and patients are unclear. But in a government-run health care chess game, both are just pawns.

The small, independent medical practices have long dominated the medical landscape. But increasingly, doctors are giving up their independence to join larger groups or hospital systems, often getting help with back-office functions like billing and insurance negotiations while staying in their old offices and seeing the same patients.

The idea is that by teaming up, doctors and hospitals can avoid repeat tests and offer the best possible care at the lowest price. It's a notion that has long been percolating in the healthcare field. They're sensing that change is necessary, and they want and desire and need perhaps a partnership with a health system. So our timetable to get there into accountable care and truly clinically integrated system have sped up.

Choosing between private practice and working at a hospital may be a weighty decision for doctors, but patients may not notice much of a difference.

When Did The Sub Specialization Of Medicine Begin? And When Did It Become So Compartmentalized?

The recent decline in the production of primary care physicians has been associated with a decrease in the production of general internists and an increase in the number of medical subspecialists. A significant majority of entering internal medicine residents anticipate entering a medical subspecialty. This transition in the development of the medical workforce, perceived by some as inappropriate, is analyzed in light of historical trends in the evolution of internal medicine and its subspecialties, and in conjunction with the roles played by the American Board of Internal Medicine and the National Institutes of Health.

The evidence is presented that the creation of virtually independent subspecialty departments may have been detrimental to the education of physicians and not productive of the physician-scientists they are assumed to create.

As medical scientists specialized and devoted their intellectual energies to understanding more and more about narrower topic areas, general practitioners differentiated into physicians with specific areas of expertise, devoting some or all of their work to that specific area. The first medical specialty to create its assessment board was ophthalmology in 1917. Prompted by the growth of optometry as a separate discipline, the American Medical Association and the American Ophthalmological Society established an independent board of specialists to create standards that would recognize physicians whose knowledge and skills demonstrated expertise in identifying and treating disorders of the eye.

Also, the new specialties can benefit both patients and physicians. However, a proliferation of specialties without adequate justification may simply confuse the public without creating a social good. The use of specified criteria can lead to rational decision-making that balances the potential benefit of recognizing more specific expertise to the detriment of fragmentation of the profession. This approach extends beyond traditional specialization, which requires formal training, to the recognition of new areas of expertise that physicians gain while in practice — that is, focused practice.

What About Medicare And Medicaid And How They Are Funded

Medicare is an entitlement program that provides health insurance to persons aged 65 and older or to those with disabilities without regard to income. Medicaid is health insurance available to certain people and families who have limited income and resources. It covers an estimated 58 million people. Medicaid is overseen by the federal government, but each state establishes its eligibility standards and determines the scope of services. States also set the rate of payment for services, and administer their own Medicaid programs.

Like Medicare, Medicaid is overseen by the Centers for Medicare and Medicaid Services of the Department of HHS.

The Medicare program, enacted in 1965, provides seniors with health insurance coverage comparable to that available to non-elderly and non-disabled Americans in the private sector. It includes hospital insurance (Part A), supplementary insurance (Part B) to cover outpatient and home health services as well as physician visits, and prescription drug coverage (Part D). Seniors also have the choice to enroll in private plans (Part C), called Medicare Advantage, to cover their services. The Medicare program covers 44 million people, 37 million seniors, and 7 million disabled Americans. It is funded by Federal payroll taxes, general tax revenues, and beneficiary premiums. Medicare is administered by the Centers for Medicare & Medicaid Services (CMS).

The Medicaid program is jointly funded by the federal government and states. The federal government pays states for a specified percentage of program expenditures, called the Federal Medical Assistance Percentage (FMAP). States must ensure they can fund their share of Medicaid expenditures for the care and services available under their state plan.

States can establish their own Medicaid provider payment rates within federal requirements, and pay for services through fee-for-service or managed care arrangements. To change the way they pay Medicaid providers, states must submit a State Plan Amendment (SPA) for CMS review and approval.

Why Can't We Buy Health Insurance Like Auto Insurance?

During the debate over health insurance reform, you'll occasionally run into the idea that health insurance should be provided more like auto insurance. After all, in most states, everyone has to have auto insurance, so everyone's covered. If you have a decent driving record, you'll have lots of choices among providers; and most people can find the minimum required insurance, even if it's in a high-risk pool.

If the market works for auto insurance, why not health insurance? The answer is simple: People and cars are different. We (rightly) value them differently. And the market can't account for that difference. Here's why:

First, car insurance is a very restrictive form of catastrophic coverage. It doesn't cover the everyday items that keep cars running, like oil changes; nor does it cover mechanical breakdowns, even when they cost you a fortune. You can put off an oil change, and eventually, your car will break down, but your auto insurance won't help you then. It only comes into play when you hit someone/something, or they/it hit you.

Your health is different. Your body can break down in numerous ways – cancer, pneumonia, or a collision with a bus, for example. To be effective, health insurance has to cover both preventative and catastrophic care, because the two are inextricably connected. People will put off a yearly check-up if insurance doesn't cover it. And when small health care problems go unnoticed or untreated, they become full-blown problems that cost a great deal more to treat in an emergency room.

Health insurance reform is about ensuring everyone has more than catastrophic coverage or the emergency room to rely on — because it's healthier and cheaper for everyone, and ultimately better for our communities and our economy. If everyone can easily access and afford preventative care, that means fewer expensive trips to the emergency room.

A better analogy for health insurance is the local fire or police department. It doesn't matter how much you earn, or how high up the social ladder you are; you get the same fire engine. Maybe you can afford better home monitoring and security if you are wealthy, but you don't get better fire engines or faster patrol cars. And you don't get a bill in the mail when a fire is put out, or a burglar is caught.

When Were The First Hospitals Created?

Pennsylvania Hospital happens to be the first hospital created. It is was founded in 1751 by Dr. Thomas Bond and Benjamin Franklin "to care for the sick-poor and insane who were wandering the streets of Philadelphia." At the time, Philadelphia was the fastest growing city in the 13 colonies. In 1730, the population numbered 11,500 and had grown to 15,000 by 1750 (the city continued to grow, and by 1776, its 40,000 residents made Philadelphia the second largest English-speaking city in the British Empire).

At the time, colonial America's urban centers were far healthier than their European counterparts. Nevertheless, the Philadelphia region, according to city leaders of the day, was "a melting pot for diseases, where Europeans, Africans, and Indians engaged in a free exchange of their respective infections." Faced with increasing numbers of the poor who were suffering from physical illness and the increasing numbers of people from all classes suffering from mental illness, civic-minded leaders sought a partial solution to the problem by founding a hospital.

The idea for the hospital originated with Dr. Thomas Bond. Born in Calvert County, Maryland, Bond, a Quaker, moved to Philadelphia as a young man. In 1738, to further his medical education, he went abroad to study medicine in London. While in Europe, Bond spent time at the famous French hospital, the Hotel-Dieu in Paris, and became impressed with the continent's new hospital movement. Bond returned to Philadelphia in 1739 and two years later was appointed Port Inspector for Contagious Diseases.

Chapter 2

THE NERVOUS SYSTEM
– CENTRAL TO GOOD HEALTH

When we were first conceived, the first thing created in all of us was the brain. Next, it was carefully encased in a bony hard substance called the cranium. Afterwards, the spinal cord, an extension of the brain was created, and that too was encased in a protective layer called the vertebrae or spinal column.

The next part to be developed in-utero was the spinal nerve roots, which are extensions of the spinal cord. Ultimately, those spinal nerve roots create spinal nerves which are surrounded by embryonic tissue. The brain is then stimulated by the embryonic tissue via the super highway called the nervous system. It was then and only then, that the other systems in the body developed.

You see the nervous system is what controls all the systems in the body. If you were to look up nervous system in the Webster's Dictionary, you would find it defined as the following: "The master control system of the body that controls all other systems of the body."

The nervous system consists of three different areas. The first is the brain. It is the originator of the messages that are needed to be distributed to all the cells, tissues, organs, and systems of the body.

The second part of the nervous system is the spinal cord. Think of it as the super highway of the nervous system. It is a complex system which has routes to every aspect of our body.

The third part of the nervous system is the spinal nerve. Think of this as an exit off the main highway. Without these exits, you can never really get to a specific destination.

The brain weighs only 3 pounds. It needs only the energy of a 10 watt bulb, yet the functions of the brain are truly staggering. The brain is so complete and complex in its function that you would need two buildings the size of the Empire State Building to house today's technology that would rival the power of the brain.

Let me explain further. The brain can perform billions of operations simultaneously. Billions! A computer can only perform one task at a time. A computer can perform the task at astounding speeds, but it can only perform one function at a time. Therefore, in order to have the computer be able to replicate the full capacity of the nervous system, you would need a massive system enabling the computer to perform complex tasks; billions of them at the same time. That is why the nervous system is called the master control system of the body. It controls all other systems. Without it, you could not survive.

Here is another way to emphasize the importance of the nervous system. If you cut the nerve to the lungs, how would the lung know what to do? Think of the lung as an appliance, and the spinal cord is the circuit. If the circuit breaker isn't allowing energy to flow into the outlet that supplies the appliance, the appliance is not going to work. It's the same with the cells, tissues, organs, and systems of the body.

The Workings of the Nervous System

Intelligence flows through every cell in the body. This intelligence is referred to by chiropractors as Innate Intelligence. Without this intelligence, there would be no order and no divine collaboration within our body.

There is an internal divine guidance that guides all the functions of the body. It knows exactly what substance to produce at the exact time needed. The neuronal connections within our body are truly staggering. In the brain alone, there are more possible connections than there are possible combinations of phone lines within the Unites States. Just imagine that number!

So what prevents our body from doing its thing? What prevents this splendid orchestra from playing its tune called health?

Interference with the nervous system can have serious complications. Think about this for a moment. If I'm on a phone and I'm giving you very detailed instructions on how to get from point A to point B, and all of a sudden your phone begins to break up, will you be able to accurately get the directions you need to get to your destination? Now, this is not because you are incompetent. It is simply due to the fact that there was a break in your communication with me.

The key is to maintain 100 % communication within every aspect of the body. The researchers are just beginning to understand that there are mechanisms within our body that are trying to communicate something very important. One example is the fever. At first fever was regarded as something that needed to be stopped. We now know that it is designed to throw off the foreign invaders.

How did we react to fevers just 10 years ago? We pushed fever reducing substances down our children's throats, and we bought into it. There are so many examples of this type of message scrambling that we do to ourselves, be it emotionally, physically, nutritionally, etc. Misunderstandings take place all the time. That is why I'm writing this book -- to at least give you a basic understanding of your body and what you can do immediately to bring it the next level. You have a very sophisticated body which needs a sophisticated understanding on how to provide it with the essential care it needs.

If the entire nervous system is fully functioning and fully interactive, with all the cells, tissues, organs, and other systems in the body, then the body can effectively and efficiently respond appropriately to dangerous conditions in the body. However, if the nervous system is not functioning properly, then you will find that it will create an imbalance, or lack of ease also called dis-ease.

The mindset that we have in regards to our bodies must be changed. Do we just get by in a world that is cruel, or is life a miracle, and the body that I am in the temple of my soul? Do we have reverence for our bodies? Again this book is a wake up call for you to realize that there is so much in all of us to stimulate health -- so much potential. Unfortunately, most of the time, through ignorance, the body is just wasted away.

In coming chapters you will realize that our bodies can be the most amazing source of super immuno-stimulation and yet it can also be the greatest source of disease creation. The great researcher Gary Null, has advocated that health can be broken down into 25% nutrition, 25%

exercising, and a whopping 50% mental attitude. If we have certain expectations and we believe them with certainty, those expectations will manifest in the physical world. In other words, you truly become what you think about, good or bad. What we must remember is that the intelligence that created us at conception still flows through every cell in our body today, and we must honor that.

I tell my patients that the body is providing us with signals, and we can not ignore those signals. Again, I will stress one thing; I or any other chiropractor, doctor or naturopath does not cure anything or anyone! The body does the curing. Think about it, you see all these doctors that boast about their achievements with patients, yet if they truly understood the innate intelligence that flows through us all, he or she would humbly become obedient to that intelligence and do everything they could to align themselves with the principles of health.

The body can either be used in its amazing splendor or it can be abused, and if it is abused, you will suffer with the consequences of natural law. So if we are to attain incredible levels of health, we must first start with an equivalent level of gratitude for our body and respect for it. When you realize that you have a choice, to make this life what you want of it, to carve out of life what you want, to create a magical life full of passion, vibrancy, and possibility, then you must be grateful for what you have. Think about it. There are so many things for which you can and should be grateful. The body that you are in right now is doing everything it can to support you at this very moment. It is there to serve you. So today I want you to decide that from now on, you will no longer look at your body as something that deserves a candy bar or a soda. Think of it as one of the finest, exotic cars in the world, one that deserves and should receive only the best fuel.

If you owned a $100,000 race horse, you would train it constantly. You would feed it the best food possible. Why? Because you paid all that money and you expect to get a return on your investment. Well what do you suppose you and your health are worth? How much would you be willing to pay for a liver transplant? How much for a kidney transplant? How much for a heart transplant? How much for your hearing? How much for your vision? Can you now see how valuable and priceless you really are?

Realize that you are a gift from your creator, and that you are here for a reason. That you are here not to be a wandering generality, but a meaningful specific, a person destined to achieve something worthwhile. You can't attain your heart's desires without the spark of energy derived from a true level of health and well being. Begin today with a new appreciation that your life demands true energy, not just bouts of it. It deserves a level of health that rivals the idea you once thought of as acceptable.

The Spine

The primary component to chiropractic is, of course, the spine. It is the spine, which for the sake of our discussion is made up of the spinal cord and vertebrae that is central to the science of chiropractic.

By giving you a little anatomy lesson on the spine, it will help you understand how and why chiropractic makes so much sense to those of us who have adopted this practice as our lifelong vocation.

The spinal column is a row of bones that encircle the spinal cord. The spinal cord is the central component of the central nervous system which transmits signals throughout the body. Some people assume that the spinal cord and nerves only transmit signals about touch and pain.

It is believed that the nerves signal the brain when you touch something hot, pain then registers in the brain and you quickly remove your hand from the iron. This much is true, but there is so much more information that the nervous system communicates to the brain and other organs in the body.

In chiropractic it is known that every area of the body is supplied with information that comes from the nerves. When there is no static, if you will, what chiropractors refer to as subluxation in the message transmitted, every organ can function at its fullest capacity. That is the number one purpose of chiropractic – to remove static from the message signals and open the channels for the body to mend and heal using its own innate intelligence.

Regions of the Spine

The spine can be broken down into three key regions. There is the cervical spine, thoracic spine, and lumbar spine. There is also a fourth area referred to as the sacral region. The sacral region, however, only has two bones: the sacrum and the coccyx. These are at the bottom of the spine and extend into the pelvic area.

Within the top three regions of the spine, the vertebrae are all assigned numbers. So when there is a misalignment in a particular vertebra, the chiropractor may explain to the patient that there is a subluxation caused by the misalignment of the C4 vertebra. This would mean the 4th vertebra from the top, or the 4th vertebra in the cervical spine, is misaligned.

A patient who has a blockage or misalignment in the C4 vertebra could actually be seeing the doctor about their hay fever and not necessarily back pain. That is because the nerves that extend from the C4 vertebra are responsible for messages sent to the nose, lips, mouth, eustachian tube, and mucous membranes. Often a misalignment here manifests itself as hay fever, postnasal drip, adenoid infections, and other upper respiratory symptoms. There can even be problems with hearing by a misalignment of the C4 vertebra.

Every nerve that extends from the spinal column is responsible for an organ, function, or performance of some part of the body. This includes the obvious organs such as the sensory capabilities of touch, which goes literally to every part of the body. A complete body map shows this radial effect. If you were to envision an outline of the body and create lines from the center where the spine would be located, drawn out to each extremity, then you can see how the nerves and protective vertebrae are assigned to those areas within the body. You can also see clearly, then, how if the vertebra meant to protect the nerve gets pushed out of place, even slightly, how that can have an impact on the nerve signals that go out from that region of the spine.

This idea of the vertebrae being labeled and the corresponding nerves reaching out to all areas of the body is not exclusive to chiropractic. The medical field also recognizes the anatomy and what it means to have something out of alignment. Where mainstream medicine and chiropractic differ, is in the way it is treated and in recognizing the full impact of the misalignment.

How the Spine Moves

The spine is able to bend and move and return to its "s"-like shape without incident or injury because of some of the soft tissue that works with the bony vertebrae. There are two types of soft tissue that are important in helping the spinal column protect the large central nerve, the spinal cord.

An inter-vertebral disk can be found between each vertebra. This disk helps absorb shock as the spine bends and twists during normal movement and activity. It also protects the vertebrae and spine from excessive shock. You don't think about that as you bend down to pick up a toy off the floor, because everything is in its proper place. You can even bend and twist to one side to grasp the toy that slid under the chair. Still no problems. However, if you were to have a deterioration of that disk or if it were to have slipped out of place even a little, there could be a grinding of the bone and a pinching of a nerve, and you would feel pain.

This type of back injury or painful condition is probably the number one reason people visit a chiropractor. Luckily, there are so many more health reasons that keep them returning to the chiropractor to maintain their overall health.

The second type of tissue is the facet joint. This allows for limited movement of the spine. The facet joints regulate movement so that routine movements are restricted to the point that they will not injure the spinal cord. The body, with its innate ability to heal, was created in a way that protects the most vital organs. The ribs protect the heart and lungs. The skull protects the brain. Then there is the spinal column to protect the spinal cord.

Misaligned Vertebrae

Every nerve in the body that radiates from the spinal cord supplies important information to the area of the body for which it is responsible. The example of the C4 vertebra being out of alignment is just one of literally hundreds of slight misalignments that can cause subluxation, that interference with the nerve signal, and result in some kind of ailment.

In the medical world, a patient visiting the doctor for indigestion or heartburn will almost immediately be prescribed some kind of antacid to ease those uncomfortable symptoms. For some people, this kind of quick fix may be okay for a while. After all, we all want to get rid of painful discomfort as quickly as possible. The problem with this treatment is that it doesn't cure the problem. It hardly even addresses the problem and certainly neglects the real cause of the problem. How can the body ever hope to heal itself if medications are momentarily quieting the symptoms?

Symptoms are there for a reason. The body, in its wisdom, has to let the brain know something isn't right. If we just quiet that inner voice with a medication, it's like telling someone to stop talking when they see you are about to get hit by a car. They are trying to give you an important message, but if you ignore it long enough, you will eventually have to deal with a much bigger problem.

When there is a symptom related to the stomach, it can often be traced back to the T6 vertebra. It is from this area that stomach problems and the body's ability to correct them transmit. The nerves in the T6 region could be experiencing some kind of interference. Removing that blockage through an adjustment of the spine will open up the lines of communication to the stomach and allow the problems in that region to be corrected naturally.

This simplified lesson on the anatomy of the spine is meant to illustrate the complex nature of the spinal column and the central nervous system. It is not quite as simple as explained here. There are so many minor misalignments that can impact one region of the body. Likewise, there are many different ways in which symptoms manifest themselves that it isn't always easy to pinpoint just what the real problem is. Back pain can often originate in the stomach and vice versa.

Headaches can be the symptom for so many other ailments that may start out in a completely different area of the body. The complexities of this whole system is what chiropractors study for years so that they can perform the right diagnostic tests and begin the correct treatment for any specific ailment.

Chapter 3

HEALTHY ORGANS

The Heart

How is the heart such a miraculous muscle? Synchronicity could be a way of describing the heart. It is an elaborate mechanism of supplying the entire body with blood and one that marvels scientists to this day.

On average, your heart beats 100,000 times a day without you having to think about it. It doesn't take any time outs; it doesn't go on vacation. It does its job every second of the day. Also, on average the heart pumps over 6,000 quarts of blood a day through a network of vessels that span close to 60,000 miles throughout the body. In an average life span, the heart will beat over 1 billion times. The heart's valves are made up of tissue so delicate that they are thinner than tissue paper, yet this muscle is the strongest muscle in the human body.

It is important to remember that the heart is a muscle. A muscle that is not used will whither away and atrophy. Again, you don't have to think about all this, it happens automatically. When you go to bed your heart rate goes down to conserve energy so as to rebuild and renew itself.

All of this ingenuity and it only weighs between 9 and 11 ounces! The whole point of the heart is to pick up oxygen from the lungs and supply it throughout the body. It's that simple.

The Lungs

Twenty thousand breaths are taken every day without our conscious awareness of it. We breathe in and out to provide oxygen that constitutes around 300 gallons of air, or 90 gallons of pure oxygen. Our lungs are an amazing example of coordination at it's finest. The lungs are needed to provide oxygen to the cells in which the heart circulates the oxygenated blood thereafter. This process is done by allowing the diaphragm to contract causing the lungs to expand.

When you exhale, the relaxation of the muscles takes place, and the air is released out of the lungs. When you inhale, the diaphragm and the intercostals muscles contract. This allows the chest cavity to expand. This in turn causes the lungs to expand. This causes a change in the pressure inside the lungs allowing air to enter the lungs. When you exhale the diaphragm and intercostals muscles relax, causing the pressure inside the lungs to be greater than the pressure outside, which releases the air out of the body.

During this entire process of air exchange and release, the body, upon inspiration, absorbs the oxygen from the air through a series of capillaries called pulmonary capillaries. These capillaries are very small vessels located in the alveoli of the lungs, the smallest aspect of the lung itself. Initially during inspiration, the hemoglobin in the red blood cells has attached to it carbon dioxide which must be released. This process takes place by oxygen entering into the air, which then binds with the hemoglobin of the red blood cell, causing the release of the carbon dioxide. The carbon dioxide is released through the lungs via the alveolar air sac.

Thus the primary function of the lungs is to maintain high levels of oxygen within the blood, and to remove carbon dioxide from the blood. This amazing process is carefully regulated through an elaborate system within the nervous system. Within this system, every aspect of the breathing process is closely monitored at all times to make sure that oxygen is being bound and carbon dioxide is being released. Mind you, this process is taking place every second -- on average 20-30,000 times a day. It is something we simply take for granted.

The Purpose of the Skin

The skin, although very thin, is the largest organ of the body. This integument is designed to protect the body as well as excrete toxins from the body. There are three primary areas by which the body excretes toxins via sweat. It is through the armpits, the groan area, and behind the knee.

This system also allows for regulation of temperature to take place via the blood supply to the superficial aspect of the tissue. Toxins are released through the skin when there is opportunity to do so. Too many products are being used today that interfere with our body's natural ability to release toxins from the body.

The skin is an amazing system. As the largest organ, it comprises 16% of our body weight. The skin serves many functions. It is designed to protect us from infections due to injury. It serves as a protective coating from the effects of ultraviolet through the production of melanin which it produces upon exposure to sun. Vitamin D3, the precursor to

Vitamin D, which is essential for the formation of healthy bones, is found in melanin.

Skin also acts as a temperature regulator during hot and cold conditions. It does this through a staggering supply of blood that runs along the superficial layer of the skin. In fact, in hot climates blood flow to the skin can be as much as 7 times higher as is normal, while during cold conditions blood flow is almost undetectable. This system allows the transference of heat to the surface when it is needed to remove heat through conduction, convection, and radiation.

The skin also acts as a protective border. It is in a sense part of the immune system, able to identify foreign invaders. It then stimulates the brigade and creates a cascade reaction thus stimulating the body's ability to protect itself from its environment.

Let us not forget that the skin, also allows us to communicate with the world through its extraordinary sense of touch and feel. It also responds to sudden changes in our emotions, and is the body's main organ of sexual attraction.

The Liver

The liver is located along the lower right aspect of the abdomen. What is so important about the liver? First of all it is very important. You see, the liver has many functions in the body. It is connected to the gall bladder, and it is involved in the absorption of fats and fat-soluble vitamins.

The liver has a large role in protecting the body from harmful substances as blood flows into the liver via the stomach and intestines. The liver stores and releases energy as it controls blood sugar. It regulates fat storage, aids in digestion through the production of bile, and regulates blood clotting. It produces hormones in our body and filters blood. This is important especially if we are removing bacteria and poisons.

The liver also creates cholesterol, which is necessary to every cell in the body. It produces Vitamin D, and stores minerals such as iron. Again this is all done without your awareness of it. It doesn't take a break; the liver works all the time.

The Kidneys

Each of us is born with two kidneys. They are located bilaterally just below the rib cage. Each kidney has millions of tiny tubules called nephrons. These nephrons are designed to filter the blood that circulates through it.

The kidney reabsorbs important substances that are needed for normal function in the body. The main functions of the kidneys are to filter waste from the body and retain substances that are needed such as proteins, glucose, minerals, and water. As this is all done, the kidney is able to maintain electrolyte balance.

Kidneys are important for the production of Vitamin D, which is needed for the maintenance of healthy bones. It also produces hormones which regulate blood pressure, as well as producing the hormone erthyopoeitin which is designed to make red blood cells. These are just some of the things that your kidneys do for you, every day, without you having to think about it.

The Eyes

The human eyeball is a sphere approximately 4 centimeters in size. There are millions of cells that allow for the amazing feat of vision to take place. This being said, span the room, and take a look at what you see. Try to really absorb it all. As you do this you will begin to realize that you are using a sense called sight.

Sight has an amazing spectrum to it. It is able to see millions of shades of color. This perceptual system is designed to allow different shades of color and light and different shapes all to be absorbed and understood almost instantly. The eyes can see about 3 billion colors. This is almost impossible to comprehend, especially when we are so conditioned to identify colors as simply red, blue, green, yellow, black, and white. This number incidentally, comes from scientists calculating the number of colors from a hot object from red to violet. This is called the Planck Distribution named for the scientist Max Planck.

The Hands

There are 13 different muscles in the hand. There are also 27 different bones. This allows for an incredible level of precision when picking up objects, playing the most difficult piano pieces, painting a portrait, or playing sports. All of these feats require a tremendous level of skill, yet we rarely think about what movements our hands are making as we do them. We are usually just concentrating on the task to be accomplished by our hands.

The Ears

Our hearing is an amazing creation allowing us to hear the most beautiful songs, the most cherished sounds of the ocean, the voices of our parents, children, and other loved ones. We are able to hear something that can change our life forever using these two little organs in our body called the ears.

Muscles

There are 650 muscles within the human body. A staggering 650! They are designed to propel us forward and allow us to maintain our balance in relation to gravity. They protect our internal organs, as well as provide a tremendous level of strength, so much so that if all the muscles in the human body were to pull in the same direction they would be able to pull a total of 25 tons. This again is done without our conscious effort.

We may realize the magnitude of the work the muscles do when we need to exert extra strength. However, there are so many functions of the muscles we take for granted. When was the last time you consciously thought about raising your arm up to reach for something or scratch your head?

The Skeletal System

The skeletal system is made up of 206 bones. These bones are designed to protect our internal organs and to provide resiliency against forces. They allow us to walk upright.

There are many functions for the skeletal system not the least of which is the formation of red blood cells in the bone marrow. We will be talking in great detail about the utter importance that the skeletal system has on your overall well being as it relates to chiropractic. You will be very surprised indeed on the true impact that it has on all of us.

Complex movements are achieved within the skeletal system, and yet it is capable of functioning for 80-100 years without a problem. There is a great deal you can do through nutrition and exercise that is necessary to maintain the skeletal system. This is important in order to minimize any harmful spinal decay which can take place at any age if you fail to properly maintain the skeletal system.

Chapter 4

THE HEALTH MODEL
VS. THE SICK MODEL

One important and positive way that health care is changing is that it's moving from a "sick care" model to a "well care" model. What does this mean? Well, in years past, most health care was provided on a reactive basis. Meaning when you got sick, you went to the doctor; this is the "sick care" model. Today healthcare is moving toward a "well care" model, in which a proactive approach is taken instead, through an ongoing relationship with a primary care practitioner (PCP).

The Health Model (also known as the wellness model) is a theory in caring for clients and patients that take the focus from being sick to preventative care. In the wellness model, there is a strong emphasis on holistic care where the client or patient is encouraged to take part in healthy activities that create a stronger body and mind that can ward off illness, instead of relying on the traditional health system to care for a sick body. Wellness is not just a set of practices that are incorporated at the doctor's office, but rather it's a change in lifestyle.

Wellness includes care from your regular physician but also can include chiropractic, massage, nutrition, fitness and mental health care. All of these things make you a healthier person.

Health Care vs. Sick Care

Health care is wellness. It's everything that helps you move towards health and prevent problems from occurring again or even in the first place. This includes things like nutrition, exercise, whole food supplements, dental care, chiropractic care, massage, and acupuncture.

Think of it this way. Imagine a spectrum. Health is on one end of the spectrum, and sickness is on the other end of the spectrum. Your position on this spectrum can shift toward one side or the other depending on several factors. On the health end of the spectrum, the focus is on prevention and being proactive in doing things to promote and support health. On the sick end, the focus is on addressing the crisis and being reactive to the disease or illness.

Sick care is damage control. The obvious need for "sick care" is in emergency situations, such as accidents, traumas, and other life-or-death acute conditions. Management of chronic conditions like heart disease, cancer, and diabetes is also included in "sick care." The main goal of "sick care" is to stop you from getting worse. The secondary goal is to make you feel better but not necessarily correct the cause of your problem. The "sick care" model rarely focuses on moving you back towards health and preventing the problem from occurring again.

The Wellness Approach

Wellness care seeks to turn on the natural healing ability, not by adding something to the system, but by removing anything that might interfere with normal function, trusting that the body would know what to do if nothing were interfering with it. Standard medical care, on the other hand, seeks to treat a symptom by adding something from the outside - a medication, a surgery or procedure.

Wellness is a state of optimal conditions for normal function... and then some. The wellness approach is to look for underlying causes of any disturbance or disruption (which may or may not be causing symptoms at the time) and make whatever interventions and lifestyle adjustments would optimize the conditions for normal function. That environment encourages natural healing, and minimizes the need for invasive treatment, which should be administered only when absolutely necessary. When the body is working properly, it tends to heal effectively, no matter what the condition. When the body heals well and maintains itself well, then there is another level of health that goes beyond "asymptomatic" or "pain-free" which reveals an open-ended opportunity for vitality, vibrant health, and an enhanced experience of life. This is true for mental and emotional health as well as physical health. While some people may suffer psychological disorders, creating an atmosphere of mental and emotional wellness will address all but the most serious problems.

The Concepts Of Illness Behavior And Sick-Role Behavior In Healthcare

Generally, health-related behaviors of healthy people and those who try to maintain their health are considered as behaviors related to primary prevention of disease. Such behaviors are intended to reduce susceptibility to disease, as well as to reduce the effects of chronic diseases when they occur in the individual. Secondary prevention of disease is more closely related to the control of a disease that an individual has or that is incipient in the individual. This type of prevention is most closely tied to illness behavior. Tertiary prevention is generally seen as directed towards reducing the impact and progression of symptomatic disease in the individual. This type of prevention is highly related to the concept of sick-role behavior.

In present-day public health practice, which is based on population and community-based approaches with an emphasis on participation, the research from these concepts of behavior has helped immensely in clarifying critical approaches to public health. The concept of diversity in populations has been greatly enhanced through the articulation of the concepts of illness behavior and the sick role.

Researchers now have a significant body of research showing the wide variation in these behaviors with respect to all the key demographic variables. For example, there has been excellent work showing how the presentation of symptoms to a physician is highly dependent on gender, ethnic background, and other socio-cultural characteristics. Research on the sick-role concept has elucidated the issue of power and its many manifestations in doctors' offices, hospitals, and other medical settings. It would be difficult, given this literature, for a practicing health educator not to consider the role of power in patient-physician interactions.

In general, illness and sick-role behaviors are viewed as characteristics of individuals and as concepts derived from sociological and socio-psychological theories.

Illness Behavior

The concept of illness behavior was largely defined and adopted during the second half of the twentieth century. Broadly speaking, it is any behavior undertaken by an individual who feels ill to relieve that experience or to better define the meaning of the illness experience. There are many different types of illness behavior that have been studied. Some individuals who experience physical or mental symptoms turn to the medical care system for help; others may turn to self-help strategies; while others may decide to dismiss the symptoms. In everyday life, illness behavior may be a mixture of behavioral decisions. For example, an individual faced with recurring symptoms of joint pain may turn to complementary or alternative medicine for relief. However, sudden, sharp, debilitating symptoms may lead one directly to a hospital emergency room. In any event, illness behavior is usually mediated by strong subjective interpretations of the meaning of symptoms. As with any type of human behavior, many social and psychological factors intervene and determine the type of illness behavior expressed in the individual.

The Health Belief Model

The Health Belief Model (HBM) was developed in the early 1950s by social scientists at the U.S. Public Health Service in order to understand the failure of people to adopt disease prevention strategies or screening tests for the early detection of disease. Later uses of HBM were for patients' responses to symptoms and compliance with medical treatments. The HBM suggests that a person's belief in a personal threat of an illness or disease together with a person's belief in the effectiveness of the recommended health behavior or action will predict the likelihood the person will adopt the behavior.

The Health Belief Model is a framework for motivating people to take positive health actions that uses the desire to avoid a negative health consequence as the prime motivation. For example, HIV is a negative health consequence, and the desire to avoid HIV can be used to motivate sexually active people into practicing safe sex. Similarly, the perceived threat of a heart attack can be used to motivate a person with high blood pressure into exercising more often.

It's important to note that avoiding a negative health consequence is a key element of the HBM. For example, a person might increase exercise to look good and feel better. That example does not fit the model because the person is not motivated by a negative health outcome — even though the health action of getting more exercise is the same as for the person who wants to avoid a heart attack.

The HBM derives from psychological and behavioral theory with the foundation that the two components of health-related behavior are the desire to avoid illness, or conversely get well if already ill; and the belief that a specific health action will prevent, or cure, illness. Ultimately, an individual's course of action often depends on the person's perceptions of the benefits and barriers related to health behavior. There are six constructs of the HBM.

Perceived Susceptibility: This refers to a person's subjective perception of the risk of acquiring an illness or disease. There is wide variation in a person's feelings of personal vulnerability to an illness or disease.

Perceived Severity: This refers to a person's feelings on the seriousness of contracting an illness or disease (or leaving the illness or disease untreated). There is wide variation in a person's feelings of severity, and often a person considers the medical consequences (e.g., death, disability) and social consequences (e.g., family life, social relationships) when evaluating the severity.

Perceived Benefits: This refers to a person's perception of the effectiveness of various actions available to reduce the threat of illness or disease (or to cure illness or disease). The course of action a person takes in preventing (or curing) illness or disease relies on consideration and evaluation of both perceived susceptibility and perceived benefit, such that the person would accept the recommended health action if it was perceived as beneficial.

Perceived Barriers: This refers to a person's feelings on the obstacles to performing a recommended health action. There is wide variation in a person's feelings of barriers, or impediments, which lead to a cost/benefit analysis. The person weighs the effectiveness of the actions against the perceptions that it may be expensive, dangerous (e.g., side effects), unpleasant (e.g., painful), time-consuming, or inconvenient.

Cue To Action: This is the stimulus needed to trigger the decision-making process to accept a recommended health action. These cues can be internal (e.g., chest pains, wheezing, etc.) or external (e.g., advice from others, illness of family member, newspaper article, etc.).

Self-Efficacy: This refers to the level of a person's confidence in his or her ability to successfully perform a behavior. This construct was added to the model most recently in mid-1980. Self-efficacy is a construct in many behavioral theories as it directly relates to whether a person performs the desired behavior.

Limitations of Health Belief Model

There are several limitations of the HBM which limit its utility in public health. Limitations of the model include the following:

- It does not account for a person's attitudes, beliefs, or other individual determinants that dictate a person's acceptance of a health behavior.
- It does not take into account behaviors that are habitual and thus may inform the decision-making process to accept a recommended action (e.g., smoking).
- It does not take into account behaviors that are performed for non-health related reasons such as social acceptability.
- It does not account for environmental or economic factors that may prohibit or promote the recommended action.
- It assumes that everyone has access to equal amounts of information on the illness or disease.
- It assumes that cues to action are widely prevalent in encouraging people to act and that "health" actions are the main goal in the decision-making process.

The HBM is more descriptive than explanatory, and does not suggest a strategy for changing health-related actions. In preventive health behaviors, early studies showed that perceived susceptibility, benefits, and barriers were consistently associated with the desired health behavior; perceived severity was less often associated with the desired health behavior. The individual constructs are useful, depending on the health outcome of interest, but for the most effective use of the model, it should be integrated with other models that account for the environmental context and suggest strategies for change.

Preventative Healthcare

Health is a state of wholeness in which your body knows its ever-changing needs and responds to those, all on its own. Inside Out

Chiropractic believes that chiropractic care is a long-term form of preventative healthcare that maintains your body's nervous system to keep you in good health for a lifetime.

True chiropractic care in a principled practice believes that bodily health exists when the body is in a state of wholeness; it understands its own constantly-changing needs, and is able to respond to them on its own. Chiropractic care doesn't heal injuries; rather, it helps the body to engage its own incredible natural healing abilities through a long-term routine of preventative healthcare maintenance for the nervous system.

Preventative healthcare focuses on your entire nervous system: your brain, spinal cord, and every one of the millions of nerve connections throughout your body. It monitors your entire body and all its needs, to help control and coordinate the necessary responses that allow the body to learn, adapt and constantly maintain its own health and wellness.

Preventative Care Vs. Sick Care

The common healthcare model in the United States is the sick care model. It only looks at your body after symptoms of illness present, and then considers how best to treat these symptoms.

The preventative healthcare chiropractic model, on the other hand, is entirely natural, non-invasive, doesn't rely on chemicals, and looks to the root cause of your underlying health issues. It is focused entirely on correcting spinal subluxations to allow your whole nervous system to communicate better and increase the body's overall healing abilities. This improves your ability to adapt to stress and a variety of health conditions and helps to restore you to normal, healthy and optimal function. Chiropractic can restore your natural healing capability, and provide increased vitality, energy, bodily functions and overall health.

Hospitals and the Wellness Sham

Furthermore, while hospitals and health systems may preach wellness, few offer comprehensive services designed to improve your health and well-being. Rather, they pay lip-service to this essential component of health care – viewing wellness more as a marketing opportunity than a true effort to do everything in their power to minimize unnecessary and costly utilization of their medical services.

There's no surprise here, since the dominant reimbursement mechanism, the fee for service, rewards the provision of medical services – not maximization of the health of a defined population. As a result, we pay a very dear price.

How to Move from Sickness to Wellness

This can be a big challenge for some of our clients. And the reality is, moving from a sickness state of mind to a wellness state of mind is incredibly personal. It is possible to shift from a sick-care system that doles out interventions to manage the burden of chronic illness to a positive health system, focused on wellness/well-being system that minimizes unnecessary utilization by focusing on population health. However, it would require tremendous will on the part of numerous constituents to achieve such a powerful transformation.

The key to transitioning from one model to the other is time and support. When we meet a new client who can benefit from the wellness model, we address their immediate issues, and then create a positive and encouraging atmosphere that they can feel comfortable expanding into. If they've come to see us for chiropractic care, we may encourage them to support that function with a visit to one of our massage therapists or a fitness class. Treating the whole body with kindness and mindfulness is often all it takes to move a client from being "sick" to being "well."

Far short of transformational change, there are nonetheless small seeds of hope in the form of new, evolving reimbursement and delivery models, such as ACOs and medical homes that stress population health management. Unfortunately, the pace of adoption is glacial. For providers who have been burned in the past by assuming the risk for a defined population, there's little enthusiasm for doing so again.

Our Role in Changing the System

More than three decades ago, Jim Fries gave us one of the keys to healing American health care; a silver bullet. The question is whether we have the fortitude to change the healthcare paradigm, as well as accept the personal, stewardship responsibility for our health that is essential to success. Below are the roles for each of us to play:

Government: There needs to be dramatically increased spending on proven prevention programs that can be administered at a local, state, or federal level. Furthermore, there need to be greater rewards under governmental reimbursement programs for those providers who embrace risk and demonstrate their ability to reduce the morbidity of a defined population.

Consumers/Patients: We need to understand what it means to be prudent stewards of our health, and the health of our families. It is essential that we understand the role lifestyle choices make in determining our health, and how we might combat risk-factors that imperil our future. For many of us, we will need to have access to resources that will aid in this journey – particularly if we are socio-economically challenged, and thus find lifestyle change all the more difficult. As has been well-demonstrated, the social determinants of health play a profound role in wellness and well-being.

Providers: Healthcare executives need to take the moral high-ground and do the right things for the communities they serve. One place to begin is with the development of a strategic wellness plan illustrating how wellness initiatives can be integrated into the very fabric of your hospital or health system's care model. Once developed and implemented, you can then reasonably assert that you do everything possible to minimize unnecessary consumption of health care resources while maximizing the health and well-being of your patients.

Insurers/Payers: There needs to be an unremitting pressure to partner more fully with providers on the assumption of risk for the health and well-being of a defined population, thus accelerating the demise of fee-for-service medicine, and its replacement with a reimbursement mech-anism that rewards wellness.

Employers: There needs to be broader adoption and implementation of wellness programs that incorporate proven mechanisms for elevat-ing the health and well-being of an employed population. Such programs will likely involve potent incentives for lifestyle modification by those employees at risk.

Conclusion

It's time to put the "health" back in healthcare. Physicians must join with other health care practitioners whose focus is on building health and wellness and not just managing disease and illness. Drugs and surgeries target the main complaint and symptoms. But they fail to address the cause of the problems plaguing current day society. No amount of medication will address the true cause of degenerative diseases if the dysfunction within the body is not identified and restored. The irony is that the majority of the top 10 causes of death in modern society are rooted in diet and lifestyle (heart disease, certain cancers, diabetes, Alzheimer's – to name a few). These conditions may never have grown to their current epic proportions if the medical community would have continued to honor the fundamental health building values of diet and exercise.

Chapter 5

PHASES OF HEALING

In a former chapter, we have explained the chiropractic practices and how these can assist you and your system switch back to a healthy, optimal state. To comprehend better how this approach can aid in you in increasing your strength, health, and longevity, this section will be dedicated to the specific cycles of chiropractic healing. But before we jump onto this, we are going to affirm this statement-- chiropractic practice isn't a fast cure or overnight miracle. If your system is out of whack, that is the result of years of issues to reach that unhealthy condition. While the good news is that, it won't take years to regain back your health, it will take some time for sure. Therefore, you need to practice patience and devotion. Let's now explain all the cycles, one after the other.

STAGE 1-THE INTENSE INFLAMMATORY PHASE

This is the stage that urges people to pay more attention and seek some type of expert help. This could be conventional medicine methods or alternative means, when everything else doesn't manage to bring the desired effects. Why is that? Simple because this pain is governed by its own pain and discomfort. Remember previously in this report where we dispelled the misconception that chiropractic practice was painful?? Chiropractic method in its nature is not painful. What actually triggers pain is your system's reaction to painful and sore tissue under work. Some of your joints and muscles are connected to be soft. Or perhaps your overall system is painful, which is a result of your own system's hypersensitivity to pain, as your body is subject to this pain for long periods of time.

This is the stage in which we chiropractors examine our patients because at this point, it is given that the patient experiences some level of pain or signs of discomfort like swelling, itchiness, redness, loss of balance and so on. The patients that come to visit us, are not doing so because they want to improve their health, but because they are fed-up of being in pain. Their main concern is to reduce their pain and symptoms and not the underlying mechanisms or origins of their issue.

It is vital to state here that this stage doesn't just happen overnight. It took ages and many years for your system to reach such a painful status and years of mishandling and doing inappropriate moves. So, as supported in this report, healing during this initial stage requires some time and can take up to 4 months to see good results. And anticipate that you'll have to come to a chiropractor's office once or twice a week. While this may sound a bit far to the ear's of the average american who wants a quick fix, it is actually a minimal investment for your long-term health.

It should be pointed out though, that therapy will vary in regards to power and frequency, based on the following factors:

- Sex
- Age

- Height
- Weight
- The time you've been suffering from this issue
- The level you are capable of following your physician's suggestions
- The max. pain level you can tolerate
- If and whether you experience other health problems

Upon the initial consultation, the chiropractor will assess all the above parameters as well as any other relevant aspects and problems, to come up with a personalized plan for your case. Your needs and challenges of course, will be also taken into account. However, this isn't like medicine--the chiropractic approach isn't the same for everyone.

STAGE 2-THE RESTORATIVE AND CORRECTIVE STAGE

During this stage, you pain and discomfort issues will begin to subside. Your pain will become much more tolerable and while you won't feel as if you are running like a first-class athlete, you will most likely feel better and have a more positive mood. Sitting or standing will no longer be painful.

This is the point where we rely to rehabilitate strength and integrity and take off the damaged tissue that prevents the road to full and felt recovery. This a great stage as the patient starts to feel better. The energy levels of the patient start to increase and the scope of motion is restored. This is due to the fact that pain "eats" vast amounts of energy. So the logic of pain reduction to increase energy during this stage, has a point.

But there is one aspect that we need to pay extra attention to, during this cycle of treatment and this is to avoid pushing you and forcing you too early. Like most folks who get treated, you might mistakenly think that you can do everything you wish, after you've just begun to feel better. The issue is, if you push yourself too hard and do inappropriate movements, you may end up with worse pain than before, due to the fact that your initial issues that made you visit a chiropractor in the first place are still lingering in your system.

During this phase, our aim in chiropractic treatment is to concentrate our movements on the boost of spinal mobility so that the healthy physiological function is restored to your spine and nerves. You might still have to visit your physician once of week but this depends on the intensity of your condition.

Keep in mind that this correcting stage isn't a brief one, but there are other parameters and factors that can surely affect the speed of the healing progress. This can feature length of time and intensity of the issue. If, for instance, you come to the office after suffering from multiple car accidents in a row (yep, it might sound bizarre but I had a patient like this), of course, it will take much more time for the therapy to start working compared to the average patient that has poor posture problems intensified over the last few years. Some things that affect the therapy and slow down the progress are:

- Poor diet/nutrition
- Smoking
- Stress
- Improper ergonomics
- A negative mindset

We'll tackle some of these factors as we proceed with this section. (the only thing we won't address is smoking as there are countless of studies and evidence that proves the destructive effects of smoking and you don't need us to tell you so). In a later section, we will also to some basic nutrition guidelines to help speed up your recovery process. But at the moment, we are going to proceed to the next healing cycle.

STAGE III-THE MAINTENANCE STAGE

I love seeing this specific stage in a patient that visits me. This means that they have followed the treatment and there doing what they can do to restore their health and feel their best they have ever felt maybe in their life. The pain is minimized or at least kept under control.

Once the system achieves a state of health, it's necessary to maintain it. The good thing is that while you go through this phase, it's much easier to maintain your body to this healthy status. Remember that a status of perfect health, doesn't only imply lack of pain and disease-- it is a state of optimal physical, mental, and even interpersonal well-being. Once your system enjoys health, you will most probably feel the best you've felt for years.

Another advantage is that in this state of health, even if you are bothered by a spinal injury, it will recover more quickly and not many treatment sessions will be needed afterwards. Consider this: when a highly practiced and fit athlete endures an injury, he/she recovers more quickly than the average Joe (provided that the athlete doesn't push their limits to far and use the injured part more than they should). This is due to the fact they are used to conditioning practices and their systems are in optimal health already. Recovery, for this reason, is much faster.

Consider kids and the rate they recover from such injuries. This is due to the fact that our systems are wired from a very young age to recover and restore perfect health. As we grow older though and age, the rates of recovery start to slow down and we are less resistant and able to fight any health problems as quickly as young people. During the maintenance stage though, the system is loaded with more things to work with.

This stage goes more than a periodical chiropractic sessions, however. It boils down to lifetime habits and patterns. This where the majority of people begin to feel uncomfortable as this translates to more healthy diet, exercise, and a positive, stress-free mindset.

We hear many different excuses in our work (don't stress, we sometimes use these too as we are just humans). Perhaps the greatest excuse is lack of sufficient time. But, there is always some time to decide on what's vital in your life, what's your priority to achieve health. You should prioritize some things to make sure you take the matter of health in your own hands.

Nathaniel Branden, an inspiring psychologist who has authored many books about self-confidence and self-esteem, supports that the things we try to improve, are the things we already realize, while the areas that we neglect to work on, are the ones that we don't pay attention to and are beyond our control.

This also applies to our health. It is just something that doesn't occur overnight. You have to work on it every day. Think about gravity-- we'll have to walk against it every day of our existence but we are capable of doing this. Same goes for our health. Once we are armed with the necessary means to achieve it, we can easily work towards its achievement.

But there is no point on making it so complex, as many folks many times do. These are just a few queries to raise to yourself to help pave the way for health and rejuvenation.

- How can I enjoy today eating properly and working out?
- What foods can I eat that are healthy and taste delicious?
- What type of exercise or activity can I do that I enjoy doing?
- How can I fuel my system with the foods that it requires?
- Why do I have to eat properly?
- Why should I exercise today?

THE 9 KEY HABITS OF HEALTHY FOLKS

Now that you are familiar with the basic stages of the chiropractic science, we can jump to the 9 essential habits that healthy folks practice on a daily basis which are vital for your health. This information will help you take more thoughtful and life-changing decisions.

These 9 habits trigger substantial lifestyle adjustments, one part a time. Like in the case of every new change, if you push it too aggressively and fast, you will most likely burn out and come up with the excuse later that "it just didn't work out" and quit from making another attempt. In the upcoming chapters, we'll explain these 9 habits in great detail but for the moment, here are the key principles.

1. Water/Hydration

Everyday we'll joyously sip our cup of coffees and sodas. But when it comes to actually drinking glass of water, we just brush it off. We just can't force ourselves to drink it that easy. But drinking plain water is vital for our health--afterall, 95% of our systems are made of water and not coffee or a fizzy drink. Furthermore, water is able to expel toxins from our systems, and various studies have confirmed that drinking at least eight glasses of water daily can yield a substantial impact on the system's power to preserve health and fight of disorders.

2. Veggies

Some may feel like puking whenever they see veggies. But our parents weren't wrong when they told us back when we were kids to eat our veggies, especially green ones that are full of vitamins like spinach and broccoli. Increasing your daily consumption of greens is one of the wisest nutrition decisions you can make for your health. Consider this from a scientific perspective. When greens are out in the nature, they transmute light into energy, a procedure called "photosynthesis". By consuming wholesome and raw green leafy greens, you are taking this energy from the plants. We have stated "raw" here, because we are going to explain the misconception of cooked greens later on.

3. Antioxidant nutrients.

Antioxidants are the key foe of destructive free radicals, which are bad cell reactions raising daily as we age. Excessive free radicals have been connected to cancer in some studies. However, free radicals are not only triggered by the aging process as other factors like stress, injuries, or bad diet rich in processed and chemical loaded foods come into play.

Our parents would always tell us to eat our veggies and fruits and they had a point on doing so. Studies have also validated that our parents advice to eat fruits and veggies really pays off. One of the key factors that makes their consumption healthy, is the fact that they are naturally fortified with antioxidant nutrients. This a broad term with a rather simple explanation. Mary Beth Russell, registered dietician validates that Antioxidants are essentially nutrients that you consumer from your food that ensure the proper function of the cellular reactions that are supposed to happen inside your system.

An abundance of antioxidant substances in your systems, makes it more capable of fighting and eradicating inflammatory diseases like heart problems, diabetes, cataracts, and even cancer. But here is an issue. Only a very small minority of 7% of Americans consume sufficient amounts of antioxidant nutrients daily. This is a bit of surprise as antioxidants are not scarce to find--they are found in fruits, veggies, tea and even wine. As matter of fact, the more vivid color a fruit or veggie has, the more antioxidants they most likely contain. So how many antioxidants should we take on daily basis? Experts say 5 portions of fruits or veggies per day e.g a fruit for breakfast, 1-2 veggies for lunch, 1 fruit or veggie for snack time, and 1 veggie for dinner. This is an easy addition to your diet that will pay off for the years to come.

4. Healthy Oils

Even though we tend to pile on fat inside our bodies to a great degree, we seriously lack enough fatty acids that could benefit our health. Based on studies, the mean person has a lack of vital fatty acids that reaches 90%! Insufficient E.F.A intake is connected with heart and brain problems among a huge range of other inflammatory disorders. Now, that doesn't mean that you have to swallow that bottle of vegetable oil that's stored in your cabinet. Only certain oils are healthy and these are fish oils and flaxseed oils. We are going to elaborate on this further in a later section.

5. Proper oxygenation

It is important to repeatedly allow proper oxygenation of the tissues through mindful breathing methods (here is where cardio exercise can help you out). In reality, every few of us know how to breathe properly. We are going to mention the right techniques of breathing in the next sections.

6.Good Posture

A good reason why we are unable to breath properly, is because we have a wrong posture in the first place. When we stand or sit and squeeze ourselves, we place strain on our breathing canals as well, including our diaphragm and lungs. Bad posture additionally causes other issues. It puts stress in the spinal curve and this causes issues with the nervous system. It can also bear an impact in our moods also, as we'll examine later in this report.

7. Physical activity/exercise

Yep, we know that this is challenging and we all come-up with various excuses not to get ourselves moving. But whether you like it or not, exercise and physical activity in general is vital for your health. There are no excuses such as babysitting, running around doing house chores, or being too busy. What your system needs is a complete cardio workout plan which activates a very vital muscle in your system and that is the heart. You have to challenge it in positive manner to get it moving more blood and oxygen throughout your body. The more you can trigger it, the better it will work for your system.

8. Adequate sleep

It's no surprise that Americans lack sufficient amounts of sleep, every day. We are reportedly so busy being like that, that we neglect the necessity of sleeping adequately every night and complete a full 8 hours of sleep. The issue is, insufficient sleep is a vital culprit of poor health. People who don't sleep enough have a higher risk of suffering from poor immune system capacity. So besides inducing tiredness and fatigue, lack of sleep can also lead to the onset of other issues due to suppressed immunity.

9. Positive mindset

We don't want to sound like we have our head in the clouds or promote new-age stuff, but there is a point in having a positive mindset. If let's say you catch a cold and your mourn and complain about it, you will end up feeling worse. But if you work with it instead of "cursing it' and don't pay much attention, you'll recover faster, almost magically. Of course, this doesn't imply that you should go kickboxing or run a mile when you are ill. This is a signal that maybe your system need some resting time so take a break. But don't focus too much on that or you will feel worse.

By practicing these 9 lifestyle habits and believe in them, you will manifest a more healthy reality for yourself. Towards the next sections, we are going to explain these in more detail.

Chapter 6

THE TRUTH ABOUT GLUTEN

3 Tips for the Traveler Who is Unable to Consume Gluten

Food today comes with all types of substances and chemicals, making it hard to know what you're really eating. For instance, additives, butterfat, caffeine, coloring, emulsifiers, lactose, gluten, and more. Gluten, the last on this partial list, is a sticky substance that naturally occurs in some foods. Wheat is one type of food where gluten is found. So travelers with celiac disease and gluten intolerance need to be armed with some strategies for avoiding gluten. First of all, keep in mind the other gluten-rich or gluten-laden culprits. Included in this list are rye, barley, and oats which can be contaminated. In addition, be on the lookout for foods and drinks with hidden gluten. In what follows, are some tips for keeping your trip gluten free.

1. Shop for and prepare food ahead of time

Shop well ahead of your trip by visiting your local grocery store or a website dedicated to providing gluten-free products, such as the "Gluten Free Palace." You can even buy products like muffins, pretzels, bagels, etc. in bulk. Pack such items for your trip, and be sure you have extras in case you experience trip delays or extra hungry moments.

If you are traveling by air, any condiments such as dipping sauces, must be in clear containers with a 3.4 ounce maximum. The Transportation Safety Administration's website indicates food must be wrapped or in containers that can pass through the X-ray machines.

Cooking ahead is another good idea for people who are unable to consume gluten. If you prepare small portions and freeze some for traveling, you can have your own ready-to-eat gluten-free meal while traveling.

In particular, if you are traveling in a vehicle for many hours, it is wise to pack two to three gluten-free meals and gluten-free snacks and drinks to take along with you for the day. That way, you do not have to rely on stopping to eat at questionable restaurants. Be sure to take along a cooler for your food that is filled with ice or one that plugs into your car.

2. Ask others for tips

Align yourself with people with celiac disease or gluten disorders to see if they might have some good suggestions for traveling gluten free. Celiac.com is a good example of a membership forum for such individuals. Before you embark upon a trip, utilize the group forum or facebook community for information on making a journey without gluten woes.

For example, you may want to ask others for recommendations on restaurants that cater to gluten-free diets. Then you can contact these restaurants ahead of time to ensure that they will be able to cater to your needs once you arrive at your destination.

A site such as Trip Advisor.com can also offer you a starting point for the information that you are looking for. In addition to getting recommendations for appropriate restaurants, you can ask others for information on nearby grocery stores that sell gluten-free items, as well as hotels that offer kitchenettes, fridges, and microwaves. You may want to pack your own toaster though, or make sure to bring special bags to protect your food items that are being toasted or microwaved.

3. Forewarn family members or friends

If your vacation involves visiting family or friends, be sure to provide them advance warning of your dietary requirements. You may even want to send them information on your condition, and the reasons why you need to avoid gluten. This can help prevent awkward moments when you arrive, allowing that person you are visiting to ensure that he/she has taken proper precautions before and during your visit.

In conclusion, there is no reason to shy away from traveling if you plan ahead, and do some preparation.

7 Tips for Surviving Family Gatherings & Holidays When Gluten Free

One of the most difficult things about having celiac disease or sensitivity to gluten, is that many family members do not understand it. They may think you are just being fussy or following some new fad diet, especially if they do not understand the seriousness of the condition.

In what follows, are some ideas of making it easier to survive those family and holiday gatherings. These tips can also make it less awkward, and result in a more enjoyable experience for all.

1. Communicate before the gathering

Be sure to let the host, and the rest of the family who will be attending, know that you have special dietary needs to follow. Explain to them what it is, and how gluten affects you. Sometimes, it can be beneficial to give them all a patient handout sheet that explains it, as it lends more credibility to what you are saying.

2. If possible, host the gathering

If you are prepared to, you may want to host the gathering at your own home. This way, you can ensure that a completely gluten-free meal is prepared, without the risk of cross-contamination.

3. Eat before you go

If you are unable to host the event at your place, be sure to eat at home before you go to it. By eating before, you are ensuring that you will not be tempted to eat potentially unsafe foods, because of being hungry when there.

4. Take snacks and drinks along

Be sure to take along your own gluten-free snacks and drinks. If you will be drinking alcohol, be sure to research what kind of alcohol does not contain gluten.

5. Take a gluten-free dish along

You can take your own gluten-free dish to the gathering. Just be sure to serve yourself from it first, to avoid accidental cross contamination by others there. For example, the last thing you would want is for the spoon from the turkey stuffing to touch your gluten-free dish before you do.

6. Be prepared for questions

Despite communicating ahead about your condition and the importance of following a gluten-free diet, you are still likely to be questioned. It can be helpful to ensure that you have someone else there in your court, ready to support you and back you up if needed.

7. If in doubt, do not be afraid to say you cannot eat something

The host may have had good intentions of preparing a gluten-free meal for you, but unless that person is very familiar with what that all entails, do not be afraid to stick to your own food and snacks.

4 Tips for Frugal Gluten-Free Shopping

If you or someone in your household cannot consume gluten, you quickly come to realize that gluten-free products often come with a larger price tag. All you have to do is compare a bag of regular white flour to a bag of gluten-free flour at the grocery store. The gluten-free flour comes in a smaller bag and yet it costs more. It seems wrong when going gluten-free is required to keep you healthy.

Fortunately, some governments recognize this. Canada is one country that does. It offers people with celiac disease the chance to claim the extra costs, associated with buying gluten-free products, as a medical expense. In the United States, there is no specific reference on the IRS website about being able to claim the extra costs of having celiac disease as a medical expense. However, it does appear that if your medical and dental expenses are more than 7.5% of your adjusted gross income, that you can include these extra costs as a medical claim with a letter from your doctor. It's best to speak to your accountant and/or local celiac group to find out more.

Luckily, there are ways to be gluten-free and be frugal at the same time when doing your grocery shopping. In what follows, are tips for doing just that.

1. Use foods that are already gluten-free

Fruits and vegetables, meat, seeds and nuts in natural form are good examples of foods that are naturally gluten-free.

Furthermore, now you can even find gluten-free Chex cereals in your local grocery store aisles.

2. Look for deals

Just because you are unable to consume gluten, doesn't mean that you cannot continue to use coupons, or look for sales and discounts on foods that are naturally gluten-free. Many grocery stores put their meat on sale at 30% discounts when the best-before date approaches. Even some grocery stores will put vegetables such as spinach or bags of coleslaw on sale.

Sign up online for all kinds of coupons from gluten-free ones to household products, anything that can lower your overall grocery bills.

3. Substitute snacks when possible

Gluten-free snack foods such as crackers and cookies can be expensive. However, there are many snack foods found at the local grocery store, such as everyday chocolate bars, that do not contain gluten and are priced better. When determining which snack foods to substitute with, you can call the various manufacturers and find out if their products contain gluten.

4. Create things from scratch

Unfortunately, this requires more use of your time, but it can save you a lot of money. This is especially important if you like baked goods. Therefore, it can be a good idea to buy gluten-free grains in bulk, and then use them to make the flour for your baked goods. But be sure that you are not buying in bulk at the bulk bins, as the food in there could be cross contaminated.

A note of caution: There is an exception to #4. If you only bake occasionally, it may actually be less expensive to buy the occasional gluten-free mix. This is because gluten-free baking takes some practice, patience, and trial and error, so you very well could end up making more costly mistakes when baking from scratch, if you do not do it very often.

What does a Gluten-Free Diet Entail?

Gluten is found in items that contain wheat, barley, and rye. It can also be found in oats that have been cross-contaminated. Knowing this can be somewhat helpful when figuring out which food items may or may not be appropriate if you are on a gluten-free diet.

Unfortunately, there are also many sources of hidden gluten, such as in some sauces and salad dressings. Although manufacturers are required to disclose ingredients such as peanuts and wheat (the latter of which contains gluten), they do not need to disclose barley, rye, and the other hidden sources of gluten. Not surprisingly, there are also no requirements for manufacturers to list the word, "gluten," on their labels. You have to learn how to read food labels properly to identify possible sources of gluten.

What is interesting to note is that the term "gluten free" can be used in the U.S.A. when a product contains less than 20 parts per million (ppm) of gluten. This is the level found to be where most celiacs do not experience symptoms or experience further damage to their intestines.

Here is a list of some naturally-occurring foods that are allowed in a gluten-free diet:

- Fruits and veggies
- Eggs
- Meat, fish and poultry that has not been coated with bread crumbs or made in batter.
- Most dairy
- Unprocessed seeds
- Unprocessed beans
- Unprocessed nuts
- Amaranth
- Buckwheat
- Quinoa
- Some rice

Here are foods that you can almost guarantee are made out of wheat, and therefore contain gluten:

- Flour (white, whole wheat, bread)
- Pasta

Here are other terms that you may not recognize but most certainly mean the presence of gluten:

- Kamut

- Bulgur
- Spelt
- Durum
- Malt
- Semolina
- Seitan
- Triticale
- Einkorn

Gluten can be found in a number of foods, including the following:

- Broths
- Canned soups
- Some candies and chocolates
- Soya sauce
- Hot dogs
- Processed foods
- Some medications, vitamins, and supplements
- Cereal

Of course, these are not comprehensive lists, but it gives you an idea of how many food items contain gluten. Fortunately, though, there are still many food items that do **not** contain gluten, or are below the threshold of 20 ppm. The surest way to find out if gluten is in a food item is to contact the manufacturer directly.

The key is to be patient as you learn and build your knowledge of what you can and cannot eat. It is normal to make some mistakes when beginning to follow a gluten-free diet. However, you can take comfort knowing that your health is only going to get better here on out.

5 Tips for Gluten-Free Dining in Restaurants

If you are unable to eat gluten, dining out poses its own challenges. First of all, you are trusting that the restaurant you have chosen really knows about gluten-free cooking and baking, and has taken all precautions to prevent cross contamination in a kitchen also being used to cook items composed of gluten.

Furthermore, if you are newly unable to eat gluten, you may feel nervous in making your needs known, but you will quickly learn that it is important. The better you get at communicating your needs, the less nervous you will be.

Here are some tips to make gluten-free restaurant dining a possibility:

1. Do your homework before you leave home

You can reduce your stress if you are prepared before you go out to a restaurant. There are a number of things you can do to prepare. These include:

- Look into restaurants associated with the Gluten-Free Restaurant Awareness Program (GFRAP). This program helps restaurants learn what it means to be gluten-free, about the safe preparation of foods, and more.
- Speak to the chef before you go to the restaurant to see if/how he will accommodate your dietary needs. Be sure to call when it is less busy in the restaurant, so that he can give you his undivided attention.
- Whenever possible, view the menu before going to the restaurant. Some restaurants post their menus online. In fact, many national restaurants such as Chili's and Ruby Tuesday post their gluten-free menus online. If the restaurant you are

considering does not have one online, you can always ask them to fax or email it to you. You can then search for gluten-free menu items, or find non gluten-free menu items that could possibly be prepared in a gluten-free manner by the chef.

2. Never go out when you are extremely hungry

Mistakes are more likely to occur when you head to a restaurant on an empty stomach. Be sure to eat something light before you leave home, and to bring snacks along. For example, the rest of your table may be eating breadsticks while they wait for the meal to arrive. You can safely eat some of your gluten-free snacks during this time.

3. Explain the seriousness to your server

It is very important that you be polite to your server, while emphasizing that you cannot have gluten. It can be helpful to explain it as having a "severe allergy" or "severe reaction" to gluten. Most people are aware of the seriousness of peanut allergies, and hearing the words "allergy" or "reaction" can validate that this is also serious. Fortunately, more people are becoming familiar with hearing about those who have gluten sensitivities.

If your server does not seem to understand what you are explaining, ask politely if you can speak to the chef.

You may want to carry a "restaurant card" with you, which you can provide to the chef. It can include what foods items you cannot eat (things with wheat, rye, barley, and oats), and those that are safe. www.CeliacTravel.com/cards/ is one website where you can download a free restaurant card in several different languages (this could be helpful depending on the type of restaurant you are visiting).

4. Do not be afraid to ask questions

Initially, you may feel fearful to ask questions, but all it takes is one bad food experience in a restaurant, and it can be a good reminder of the need to be assertive and clarify menu items.

You want to ask questions such as what the ingredients are in a menu item, what the preparation methods entail, and what precautions the kitchen staff take to ensure cross contamination does not occur. For example, cross contamination could occur if the same spoon is used to handle spaghetti for another customer's order, and then used for mixing your fresh salad dressing.

5. If you are served something inappropriate, say something

A very good example is if your burger comes to you and it is resting on a bun (that is not gluten-free). Because the bun has touched your burger, it has been contaminated with gluten, and it is not safe for you to eat. Therefore, you need to become comfortable telling servers in a polite manner. You will need to remind them that you will need a whole new burger made, because simply removing the bun is going to result in a severe "reaction."

Gluten Is Not Only Found In Food

The inability to consume gluten can cause a whole host of health issues. Most people are aware that gluten is found in items like certain flours. Wheat, rye and barley-based flours all contain gluten, but food is not the only thing you have to pay attention to if you are on a gluten-free diet.

You may find some of the other items, that contain gluten, quite surprising.

Things to watch out for:

One of the key issues, when being gluten free, is being able to detect products that may contain gluten. Reading labels on every item you consume is important. In many cases, the gluten is identified in the inactive ingredient (binders and fillers) list, but it's a matter of learning what those ingredients are.

3 non-food groups of items, that may include gluten, include:

1. Medication (prescription and over-the-counter)
2. Vitamin and mineral supplements
3. Cosmetics and toiletries

Medication can contain gluten, which is used to keep the tablets together and is also used as a filler in capsules. In most cases, it is not listed in the ingredients as "gluten" because the gluten is a part of another product like "maltodextrin." In addition, terms like "pregelantized starch," "dextrin," or "dextrate" are some other common compounds used in medication that also contain gluten. The Food and Drug Administration (FDA) does not require drug companies to list gluten as an ingredient. A good rule of thumb is to speak to your doctor or pharmacist to make sure that your medication does not contain gluten. If gluten is in a medication that you have been taking, your doctor may need to prescribe a substitute medication without gluten.

Vitamin and mineral supplements often contain gluten for the same reasons you find them used in medication. Once again, it is used as a binder or a filler, and is usually a part of another ingredient that may be listed under inactive ingredients. Supplements have to label their ingredients too, but laws proving their safety or efficacy are much more lax than drugs. It is therefore suggested that you look into *supplements produced by a company that follows the Good Manufacturing Practices (GMPs) established by the FDA, as this is meant to guarantee that you are getting what the label claims.*

***Cosmetics and toiletries** can be a danger to people that have celiac disease or non-celiac gluten sensitivity. Therefore, if you are completely cutting gluten out of your life, you should also consider checking all of your cosmetics to ensure that they are free from gluten binders. Gluten is usually only an issue if you ingest it so you should avoid any lipsticks, lip gloss, lip balms, toothpaste, or mouthwash that contain gluten. You would also want to choose gluten-free shampoos if there is the possibility of getting shampoo in your mouth when you rinse your hair.*

A good rule of thumb is to ask someone. Ask your pharmacist. Call the manufacturer and ask. Be persistent in getting the answers you need. If you are trying to live a gluten-free lifestyle, then it is important that you know what you are putting in your body!

5 Ways to Help Your Child Adopt a Gluten-Free Diet

Whether your child is diagnosed with celiac disease or gluten intolerance/sensitivity as an infant or as a teenager, it is important to begin teaching your child as soon as possible what it means to be gluten-free and why it is so important. Part of this teaching includes helping your child learn how to adopt a gluten-free diet.

In what follows, are some tips to help you do this:

1. Teach your child how to read labels

At any age, you can teach a child that every food item has a label on it, which contains ingredients and nutrition information.

Before children can even read, they are perceptive enough to learn how to recognize words. You can teach them how to recognize certain words such as "wheat" or "rye," for example. These are two of many words that indicate the food item contains gluten.

As children get older, you can introduce more gluten-containing words to them.

2. Be positive

One of the worst things you can do is to express your negativity or frustration, that comes along with a gluten-free diagnosis, to your child. If you are feeling negative, then be sure to speak with your spouse or another trusted adult.

You do not want to make your child feel guilty with the extra expenses that can accompany a gluten-free diet. You also do not want to make your child feel that somehow he is to blame for the extra preparation and time that is required when planning everyday meals, traveling, or family get-togethers.

3. Include your child in cooking and baking

You can teach your child the difference between regular recipes, and those made for people who cannot eat gluten. Again, be sure to explain that some people, mainly because of their genetics, cannot tolerate gluten-containing foods.

In addition, you can teach your child appropriate ways to adapt regular recipes calling for flour by substituting safe alternatives.

If your child lives in a home where not everyone needs to eat gluten-free meals, it is important to teach how to cook, bake, and even make snacks without cross contamination occurring.

4. Teach your child that it's okay to say "no" to adults and other children

Many well-meaning adults and children will offer your child gluten-containing foods and treats. You need to teach your child that it's okay to say "no" politely as these other foods can make him sick or harm his body.

5. Teach your child that gluten is also in non-food products

Food is not the only thing that your child needs to learn about. For example, items such as lip balm, play doh, and candies can contain gluten.

5 Ideas to Help Your Young Gluten-Free Child Fit in

No child wants to feel different from his peers. It is very important to fit in, and being the only gluten-free child in the classroom can potentially result in feelings of isolation. This is why it is really important for all the adults, involved in a child's life, to help out.

Ways to do this include:

1. Education

Educate the teacher and the other classroom students about *why* your child is unable to consume gluten. You want to emphasize that it is like any other medical condition, where gluten makes your child sick and hurts the insides of his body. You may even want to relate it to peanut allergies, which most children are aware of. You also want to explain that that is why your child is unable to accept food trades.

In addition, you want to educate all of them on non-food sources of gluten such as lip balm and play dough, for example.

It is also important to educate the teacher that just being in the presence of flour for paper mache projects is not safe for your child, as are some finger paints.

2. Keep a stash

Provide the teacher with a stash of gluten-free goodies for times when your child is unable to consume food items that are being prepared as part of a class project at school, or other unexpected events.

3. Send gluten-free goodies to school on holidays

During Halloween, Christmas, Valentine's Day, and other holidays, send your child to school with yummy gluten-free cupcakes and enough for his classroom peers and teacher. This way, your child is the hero for bringing in the goodies, and the children get to experience the same kind of food that your child eats.

4. Send extra snacks along in your child's lunch

Although your child is not able to eat the food from other children, there is nothing wrong with classmates eating gluten-free foods that your child brings to school. Just like the gluten-free cupcakes mentioned above, you can also send your child to school with extra gluten-free snacks in his lunchbox from time to time. This way, he can share them with peers in his classroom. The other children then get to see that your child eats food that tastes good too, but your child stays safe in the process.

5. Purchase or prepare

Foods such as gluten-free pizza and gluten-free chicken nuggets can be purchased or prepared from scratch. These foods look like those that the other children eat, only they are gluten-free.

The more your child feels the same and others view him like he is, the more he will feel like he fits in.

3 Steps to Making Your Kitchen Gluten Free

When you learn that you can no longer consume gluten, there are many major changes that you need to make. One of those changes is setting up your kitchen so that it is safe from gluten.

In what follows, are some steps you can follow to make your kitchen safe and gluten-free for your needs:

1. Begin by getting rid of gluten-containing foods

You will need to discard, or better yet, give away the food items that contain gluten or may have been contaminated by gluten in the past.

Examples of food products that likely contain gluten include flour, bread, baking mixes, and certain sauces.

Many food items that may have been cross contaminated include baking soda and baking powder, peanut butter, jam, butter, ketchup and mustard, for example. Basically, these items become contaminated when they have come in contact with gluten-containing particles. This can happen very easily and innocently. For example, if you or another family member uses the same spoon in the flour and then the baking soda, cross contamination has occurred. Another example is if your squeezable mustard container's tip has accidentally touched a gluten-containing bun. Therefore, you will need to replace these food items with new, uncontaminated ones.

2. Replace some kitchen tools

You will not need to replace everything in your kitchen, but you will definitely need to replace certain items that are contaminated by gluten.

Examples of some of these items include:

- toaster
- silicone spatulas
- colander and other strainers
- non-stick pans with scratches
- plastic bowls that have scratches in them, plastic utensils
- wooden cutting boards, wooden spoons, and wooden bowls
- mustard and ketchup containers, etc.
- rolling pin
- muffin tins or other baking sheets with scratches

3. Clean items in your kitchen thoroughly

Some of the items that cannot be cleaned thoroughly enough to be safe from gluten have been outlined above. However, some items can be cleaned enough that you can use them again. Here are some examples:

Stainless steel bowls and pots:

Just make sure to clean them well. Also be sure to clean the lids fully.

Oven & Stovetop:

Clean the top, sides, and bottom of the oven, as well as the oven racks.

Cupboards and drawers:

Bread crumbs seem to make their way into all sorts of places, including the utensil drawers and the cupboards. Sometimes, they even get into the fridge. Take this opportunity to do some spring or fall cleaning, and vacuum up all the crumbs.

Refrigerator and freezers:

Be sure to clean up the shelves to remove any crumbs or spills. Be sure to scrub any seals.

5 Tips for a Happy Gluten-Free Halloween for your Young, School-Age Child

Does gluten-free mean that Halloween has to be something that you cannot celebrate? No, it does not. It means it is time to get creative and take control of Halloween so that gluten-free does not mean missing out on the fun.

The five tips below can help you to make sure that your child gets to spend a great day without the fear of consuming a treat that will play some awful tricks on him! On the upside, there is a considerable amount of candy that is actually gluten free! It is not as hard as you think to find some. A good rule of thumb when in doubt about something is to call the manufacturer. You can even do an online search to locate some very reputable listings of gluten-free candies.

1. Take charge

Throw your own Halloween party. If you take charge of the day, then you get to prepare the treats and have peace of mind knowing that you are preparing gluten-free treats. You can combine the gluten-free items with non candy-items like plastic spider rings, that ultimately add to the fun and overall Halloween spirit.

2. Fair trade

Stock up on gluten-free candy at home. Play "Lets Make a Deal" with your child where you trade out candy containing gluten for sweet treats that do not. You can also buy the candy back! Of course, you will have to be on the losing end of the trades to ensure a happy goblin!

3. Be the class mom

If your child's school is having a Halloween party, you want to be sure that you are present to make sure that the treats, that your child is presented with, are gluten free. Bring a big bag of gluten-free options to share with the class.

4. Make it less about the candy

Focus less on the treats, and more on the fun of getting dressed up for the big day. Make it about the decorating, and carving of the pumpkin. Take photos and then scrapbook the fun in an album, and make it a yearly event.

5. Set the rules early on

Make sure that you set the rules early on about taking candy out of the bag and eating it. Purchase the candy you are going to use for "Lets Make a Deal" together. Remind your child several times before the big day about your "deal" day.

Relax and have fun. Celebrate the month with all the things that make Halloween fun besides just the candy - crafts, pumpkin picking, pumpkin carving, and enjoying the falling leaves. Try not to stress as it will work out fine with a bit of preparation and planning!

6 Ways to Avoid Gluten Cross Contamination in Your Kitchen

It is not uncommon for one person in the family to require a gluten-free diet, whereas the rest of the family can eat a regular diet.

You then need to have a shared family kitchen, meaning both gluten and gluten-free food items are prepared there. This results in the potential for cross contamination, and needs to be avoided for the sake of the person who cannot consume any gluten at all.

Here are ways to avoid gluten cross contamination from happening in shared kitchens:

1. Set up a separate, gluten-free space in the kitchen

An example of separate space includes dedicating a part of your kitchen pantry or cupboard space to gluten-free food products and those that have not been contaminated by gluten.

In addition to food items, you can also include all your gluten-free utensils and other kitchen gadgets (ex. toaster) that need to remain separate to stay uncontaminated.

It can also be helpful to ensure you and your family has a way of knowing which baking utensils, cutting boards, and so forth are meant to be kept gluten-free, and which ones are meant for the gluten-containing foods. You can do this by using a consistent color scheme. For example, all gluten-free spatulas and cutting boards are red.

2. Label items

Unless you have the space for two refrigerators, you will have to share it. In this case, you want to label your items and teach your family members that they are not to touch those labeled with your name because contact with gluten will make you sick.

Speaking of the refrigerator, you may also want to create a separate space such as one of the shelves or the side of the fridge. Just be sure that no other foods can spill on yours when they are all in the fridge together.

3. Clean the counter

Before you begin to prepare food, be sure to clean the kitchen counter with soapy, warm water.

4. Clean the sink

Make sure no crumbs or gluten-containing foods are left in the bottom of the sink before you use it. As well, be sure to use a separate dishcloth and separate dishtowel to prevent cross contamination with food particles.

5. Allow your family or roommates to confess without repercussions if they make a mistake

If you live with an absent-minded spouse or a child, it is very likely that someone will mess up and accidentally contaminate one of your food items or kitchen items.

When this happens, it is important for them to know that they can tell you without you getting mad at them. This will ensure healthy communication, and ensure that you stay healthy.

6. Wash shared kitchen items

It is okay to share stainless steel bowls, and stainless steel pots and pans, as long as they have been carefully washed after gluten-containing foods have been prepared or cooked in them. Pay careful attention to lids, where food particles can sometimes get caught.

Gluten, Celiac Disease, & Gluten Sensitivity: What You Need to Know

You have no doubt heard of "gluten." More and more products are labeled as such on the grocery shelves, and you probably know one or more people who are following a gluten-free diet.

But what exactly is gluten anyway?

It is a mixture of proteins that are found in wheat, rye, and barley. Oats do not contain gluten, but they can be contaminated with gluten. The presence of gluten in flour gives dough its stickiness and elasticity. Gluten also helps the leavening of dough by trapping carbon dioxide gas within it, allowing the dough to rise into a nice fluffy texture.

Gluten is found in many foods such as cereals, breads, pastas, and processed foods for example, as they are made from the above-named grains. It is even found in other products such as lip balms, vitamins and supplements, and medications.

What is celiac disease and what is its relationship to gluten?

If you have celiac disease, you are unable to eat gluten. It is an autoimmune disorder, meaning your body attacks its own cells, causing tissue damage. Rheumatoid Arthritis (RA) and Diabetes Mellitus are two other examples of autoimmune diseases. In fact, if you have another autoimmune disease, it increases your risks of having celiac disease.

Normally, your body's immune system is supposed to defend it against bacteria and viruses. However, in the case of celiac disease, when you ingest gluten, this triggers your immune system to attack the gluten molecules and ultimately its own small intestine lining. This then causes inflammation and damage to the intestine, resulting in poor absorption of nutrients.

What causes celiac disease?

There are three main things including your genetics, the consumption of gluten, and a trigger of some sort. This trigger can be things like stress, surgery, or pregnancy.

What are the symptoms of celiac disease?

Surprisingly, symptoms vary with individuals, and there are many different kinds of symptoms. The symptoms can mimic lactose intolerance and irritable bowel syndrome.

Although most think of celiac disease as causing gastrointestinal issues such as diarrhea and weight loss, the truth is that not everyone experiences these symptoms.

In particular, **adults** tend to have less of these gastrointestinal symptoms, but other symptoms such as:

1. Canker sores
2. Fatigue
3. Numbness and tingling in the hands and feet
4. Anemia
5. Osteoporosis (thinning of bones)

6. Depression
7. Joint pain
8. Headaches
9. Skin rash
10. Eczema
11. Vitamin and mineral deficiencies
12. Low blood sugar

In fact, these above symptoms are sometimes referred to as extraintestinal, meaning "outside the intestine," and there's reported to be hundreds of symptoms.

In **children**, some symptoms can include:

1. Delayed puberty
2. Bloating so the stomach looks big
3. Weight loss
4. Headaches
5. Attention deficit hyperactivity disorder (ADHD)
6. Diarrhea
7. Failure to thrive (not meeting expected standards of growth)

As already mentioned above, these symptoms are similar to the symptoms of other diseases too, so you need to see a physician to help you determine what is going on.

To complicate matters, some people with celiac disease have no symptoms at all! This is what is known to medical professionals as **"silent celiac disease"** or **"asymptomatic celiac disease."** However, damage is still occurring to their small intestines, so getting a diagnosis is important.

But how do you find out if you have celiac disease, with or without symptoms?

Your physician can request blood tests that look for specific antibodies. If you test positive for the antibodies, then an intestinal biopsy (this is where a small piece of tissue from the intestine is examined) is done to confirm that you have the disease.

It is important to note that you do not want to start a gluten-free diet until you have been diagnosed otherwise the diagnosis could be missed.

What is the treatment for celiac disease?

Implementing a strict gluten-free diet is the only treatment at this time. This allows your small intestine to recover from the damage it has been experiencing due to the exposure to gluten.

It is definitely easier to implement a gluten-free diet when you are experiencing symptoms and want to feel better. However, for those without symptoms, it is just as crucial that you stick to this diet too to prevent damage to the intestine, as well as the development of other health conditions which can include:

1. Malnutrition
2. Miscarriage
3. Possible congenital birth defects such as incomplete closure of the baby's spinal column during pregnancy
4. Decreased height in children as they grow up
5. Cancer in the gastrointestinal (GI) tract
6. Osteoporosis (thin bones)

Now that you have learned about celiac disease, another topic is worth discussing. That is the topic of what gluten sensitivity/gluten intolerance is.

You may also hear this referred to as **"non-celiac gluten sensitivity."** In 2011, a study at The Alfred Hospital in Melbourne, Australia, reported that gluten seemed to be a culprit in gastrointestinal problems in people who did **not** have celiac disease. However, this researcher has since conducted more research and now states that the existence of gluten sensitivity/gluten intolerance/non-celiac gluten sensitivity is not fully substantiated, and further research needs to be conducted.

Nevertheless, there are many people and health professionals who believe it exists, and when they follow gluten-free diets, they report feeling better. Many reputable sites such as the Center for Celiac Research recognize it as its own condition. So with this in mind, it deserves its own discussion.

Like celiac disease, symptoms in someone with gluten sensitivity or gluten intolerance can include stomach-intestinal problems such as diarrhea, bloating, pain, or constipation. Fatigue, depression, and joint pain are other symptoms that can also be seen.

How this condition differs from celiac disease, however, is that the tissue in the small intestine is **not** attacked. No antibodies can be found when a blood test is done, so there is no definitive way to diagnose it. Usually, this diagnosis is made by trying a gluten-free diet to see if symptoms improve.

Celiac disease stats for those affected are about 1%. In the case of gluten sensitivity, it is higher at about 6% of the population. People with gluten sensitivity/intolerance are at higher risk of developing celiac disease through repeated exposure to gluten.

What kind of diet do you need to follow?

Now that you have the lowdown on what gluten is, and how it is related to celiac disease and gluten sensitivity/intolerance, your next step is to take steps to remove the gluten in your diet. Even some non-food items (lip balms, for example) have to be replaced.

If you have celiac disease, it is imperative that you never eat gluten. If you do, your intestine will not be able to heal, which can lead to long-term health problems. Even if you experience no symptoms when you eat gluten, but you have the diagnosis of celiac disease, you have to stay away from gluten.

If you have gluten sensitivity or intolerance, no damage has yet been done to your small intestine, but to feel better and prevent the possibility of developing celiac disease later, you should also avoid gluten. However, some people with sensitivity or intolerance may cheat and eat gluten-containing foods occasionally. This is still not recommended, as it may bring on your symptoms.

To conclude, people with celiac disease and gluten sensitivity/intolerance may experience many of the same symptoms. In both cases, gluten is the culprit, and avoiding it will improve your health.

You can learn more about going gluten-free by visiting (your blog, website, etc).

Chapter 7

INFLAMMATORY SYNDROME HOW TO COUNTERACT THE EFFECTS OF THIS SILENT KILLER

BATTLING A NEW EPIDEMIC

N ow that you are familiar with some of the common factors that wreak havoc on your system, let's now mention what exactly enters your system when influenced or prone to it.

The term "inflammation", is basically an immune reaction triggered by our systems to prevent any infection by bacteria or damage e.g from injuries. If we examine human history itself, we will find out several bacterial infections and disorders that spread to whole populations but people were able to vanish them. Some of these past disorders include, smallpox, influenza, typhoid fever, and bubonic plague, which are almost extinct today.

While the majority of the above bacterial illnesses have almost vanished, nowadays, we have to face a whole new epidemic. There are multiple health issues today that shave off your quality of lives and well-being like such as, breathing problems, memory issues/alzheimer's, allergies, autoimmune disorders, skin problems, and many more. All these issues that especially affect the Western population aren't caused by bacteria like in the past but from inflammation.

In the past two decades, the frequency of degenerative diseases has been constantly on the rise. Researchers have found that inflammatory disorders have been affecting Americans at an alarming rate because of poor diet habits and induced levels of stress and anxiety. The level of inflammation is at its peak has almost grown to an epidemic. Without any substantial changes to our diet and lifestyle patterns, the country will keep on suffering from diseases like cancer, heart problems, diabetes, Alzheimer's and the list goes on.

WHAT ARE THE EFFECTS OF INFLAMMATION ON THE SYSTEM

When we use the word "inflammation", we usually think of symptoms like "heat", "high temperature", "Irritation", "swelling" and pain somewhere. When a lesion gets inflamed, we can see with our own eyes the inflammation. However, inflammation is not always externally visible like that. The physical signs of "secret" inflammation do emerge but at a much later stage, sometimes when it's too late.

Chronic (long-term) inflammation leads multiple issues in our systems. All sorts of inflammatory disorders may pop up and become a population in our bodies. A person who goes through chronic inflammation, becomes exposed to further health deterioration from diseases and even aging acceleration.

DISORDERS TRIGGERED BY INFLAMMATION

There are various health issues connected with inflammation. Some of the most commonly emerging ones are numerous kinds of arthritis. Arthritis is a broad term that refers to various kinds inflammations in the joint area. Some of the most frequent/common kinds of inflammation-triggered arthritis are:

- Rheumatoid arthritis
- Polymyalgia Rheumatica
- Bursitis
- Shoulder Tendinitis
- Gouty Arthritis

Other stressing body problems targeting the bones and joints of our body, that haven't been yet confirmed to be caused by inflammation but they are still under investigation are:

- Osteoarthritis
- Fibromyalgia
- Neck and back pain (in the muscles)

Shockingly enough, the World Health Organization reveals that over 13 millions of people annually lose their lives from cardiovascular disorders. The cancer rates are also alarmingly big, with 8 millions of people losing their lives from cancer annually. Both of these dangerous disorders are caused by chronic inflammation. So in order to control the likelihood of developing such disorders, we must adopt some healthier diet and lifestyle changes.

Heart disorders separately were to blame for 25% of the deaths in the U.S last year and numbers of people affected are constantly on the rise.

Almost 50% of the deaths linked to heart disorders were a result of chronic inflammation. The numbers may seem exorbitant and unbelievable but they are shockingly true. Inflammation is a huge factor contributing to heart problems.

Based on *National Institute of Health* findings, inflammation is a very vital factor for the development of heart disease and its aggravation. The same goes for other serious and chronic health disorders like cancer and diabetes.

FOODS THAT LEAD TO INFLAMMATION

For those affected by inflammation, diets rich in carbs and low in protein intake can be destructive. As a matter of fact, we've witnessed multiple times that such high carb and low protein diets lead to inflammation while the opposite diet (low carbs/high protein intake), actually keeps inflammation under control and all the negative side effects connected to it.

Every individual organism differs from the other, and thus it is important to spot all the signs and symptoms we experience when we take certain foods. We will offer you a diet against inflammation with all the proper foods to eat later in this report, but at this point, let's delve in a few details.

Processed sugars and foods with an elevated Glycemic Index (G.I), in reality raise insulin levels and trigger an immune system response. There is a communication between inflammatory mediators (prostaglandins, cytokines), and insulin or blood sugar amounts. Studies reveal that when specific stressors emerge, insulin triggers an inflammatory reaction within the system.

Some of the worst foods that trigger an inflammatory response in the body are:

No 1: Sugar/Sweets. High amounts of sugar consumption have been associated with overweight issues, inflammation, and chronic inflammatory diseases like Diabetes Melitus.

No 2: Typical vegetable oils for cooking and baking. Oils with a high omega-6 fatty acid/low omega-3 acid ratio, also lead to inflammation.

No 3: Trans fats. These fats are typically found on junk food/fast food meals. They are also associated with inflammation, resistance to insulin, and other chronic disorders.

No 4: Non-organic milk and dairy products. Non-organic dairy products can also result in inflammation, especially in the female population, due to the hormones and allergen ingredients they contain.

No 5: Red or processed meat. Eating red and processed meat e.g corned beef cans, is also associated with immune reactions that lead to chronic inflammation within our systems. There is also a clean connection between processed meat consumption and cancer risk,

backed-up by many scientific trials.

Other types of foods suspect of causing inflammation are grains/flour, alcohol, synthetic food preservatives, and grain-fed meats. All the above foods should be avoided inf nay signs of inflammation emerge.

LINK BETWEEN STRESS AND INFLAMMATION

Going through chronic emotional, mental, and physical stress affects inflammation in the system to a very high degree. In reality, when the system is exposed stress, cortisol levels start to rise within the body.

Cortisol is specifically a steroid hormone that is produced in response to high levels of stress. This may occur from real stressful events or an unhealthy diet or lifestyle. Concerning inflammation, the stress reaction that starts to develop to relieve the body from tolerating such circumstances isn't switched off. Chronic stress is tied to chronic inflammation responses.

In fact, chronic stress has a negative impact on various body functions. For example, it raises blood pressure and hypertension eventually. Chronic blood pressure also puts blood vessels under a tremendous amount of stress. Strokes and heart failures are a common phenomenon in people suffering from chronic inflammation because of inflammatory responses triggered non-stop.

Stress can really "eat" you! Thus, it is vital to learn ways to deal with high stress levels so that you avoid chronic inflammation. Some valuable relaxation methods include:

- Mild exercise
- Yoga/Meditation
- Consuming healthy and nutrient-dense foods
- Learning ways to keep emotional tranquility
- Breathing exercises

INFLAMMATION TREATMENT OPTIONS-THE HARSH ADMINISTRATION OF ANTI-INFLAMMATORY PILLS

The protocol of treatment in response to inflammation is the prescription of anti-inflammatory medicine. The most typically administered drugs in this case are those that provide relief from pain (pain-relievers).

Not long ago, the *American Geriatrics Society* has taken off nearly all non-steroidal and anti-inflammatory drugs from their guide of suggested drugs for people 75+ who experience chronic pain. It was found out that these drugs are overly prescribed, more than necessary and this may lead to negative side effects on the health of older people. Researchers have found that commonly used pain-relievers like ibuprofen, naproxen, and aspirin are not really beneficial for those going through chronic pain. Due to the research conducted on older subjects, researchers are also seeking to examine the excessive administration of NSAIDS in younger subjects as well.

Anti-inflammatory drugs are aimed to lessen pain and discomfort, minimize swelling, and control inflammation symptoms. They are speculated to help with the development of inflammatory disorder, but they don't always function as intended. Anti-inflammatory substances for pain relief feature NSAIDS such as Ibuprofen and Aspirin. Other substances are the ones called corticosteroids (cortisone, prednisone), and numbing pain relievers.

Typically, anti-inflammatory drug substances demonstrate exaggerated side effects. For instance, the consumption of cortisone for extended periods of time can lead to serious problems with bone strength and integrity. Those experiencing asthma symptoms should also seek an alternative treatment option due to negative side effects from anti-inflammatory drugs. Many chronic takers of NSAIDS also develop stomach ulcers and internal bleeding because of the mucus development blocking attributes of these pharmaceuticals. The gastric wall is further exposed to stomach acid in those who consume NSAIDS for longer periods of time to fight inflammation.

Alternative medicine methods approach the matter of inflammation from another perspective. Instead of prescribing synthetic drugs to hinder inflammatory reactions, they suggest the use of vitamins/nutrients and lifestyle changes. While it's true that some vitamins and nutrients have powerful antioxidant and anti-inflammatory properties, they may not completely eradicate the problem. Alternative medicine adopts a more natural way to treatment of the issue as opposed to taking artificial drugs, but doesn't often consider the trigger cause of inflammation.

Further evaluation needs to be performed to find out the exact leading cause of inflammation. It's not holistic or beneficial to only treat the symptoms, but it's just as important to pinpoint the leading culprit of inflammation.

NSAIDS AND THEIR IMPACT ON INFLAMMATION

NSAIDS (Non Steroidal Anti Inflammatory Drugs) are often prescribed against inflammation. These may differ in power and lasting effects on the system. Prostaglandins are a family of chemical substances released by system cells that trigger inflammation in the system when required.

The enzyme responsible for making these Prostaglandins goes by the name "COX" or (Cyclooxygenase). It is also further divided into 2 enzymes: COX-1 and COX-2. Both of these enzymes trigger the release of prostaglandins which lead to inflammation as a result. NSAIDS actually work to block the activity of such enzymes and control the effects of prostaglandins within the system. This eventually leads to long-term inflammation control. However, prostaglandins that guard the stomach lining and enhance blood clotting are also decreased, which results in stomach ulcers and internal bleeding in the region.

NSAIDS when taken excessively, can interfere with physiological COX-1 activity. NSAIDS also hinder the cyclooxygenase pathways. COX-1 is typically produced by normal functioning. The COX-1 stays stabilized under physiological circumstances. In case an NSAID like Aspirin enters the system, COX-1 becomes acetylated and its arachidonic acid pathway is hindered. The process of acetylation is the culprit behind aspirin's anti-clotting and blood-thinning action.

One of the most frequently used NSAIDS is aspirin, which also prevents blood clotting and eventually inhibits strokes and heart failures in people with a heightened risk of experiencing these conditions. NSAIDS though interfere with the physiological activity of heart, kidneys, and stomach due to their action.

INFLAMMATION TESTING-BLOOD EXAMINATION

In those who suffer from long-term inflammation, there is an existing protein secreted by the inflammation region that travels through the bloodstream. One of the common blood tests to find out inflammation is CRP (C-reactive protein test). This test can pinpoint any heightened levels of the protein, which is considered a sign of inflammation.

In several situations when an individual suffers from chronic inflammation which leads to a serious disorder like cancer, arthritis, diabetes, heart failure, or connective tissue (muscle, joints, bones, ligaments) disease, the CRP levels are elevated. These levels are precisely detected through blood testing.

Homocysteine amounts in the blood can also be determined from blood testing. Homocysteine is an acid that is produced by the system physiologically when we consume excessive amounts of red meat. When homocysteine levels are abnormally elevated, the person is a high risk of developing heart problems, atherosclerosis, heart failure, stroke and even Alzheimer's disease.

WHAT'S THE KEY CULPRIT OF INFLAMMATION?

Researchers and medical experts keep on examining the leading cause of inflammation. With so many contributing factors and issues linked to our diets, it's no surprise that gut inflammation has a vital role to play here. We will explain the matter in more details in a later section, but at this point, we should be aware that there is a clear connection between the gut and inflammation. We will examine beyond the natural ways of treating its effects, but study the leading causes behind such symptoms.

Based on scientific evidence, Leaky Gut Syndrome may be the leading cause of many digestive tract diseases like IBS, Crohn's Syndrome, and celiac disease. It can also be the culprit behind the onset of various inflammatory disorders like asthma, allergies, arthritis, and chronic heart problems and disorders.

Practical/holistic medicine takes into consideration the triggering causes of a disorder and doesn't just provide a remedy for the treatment of the symptoms. It is vital to examine all these triggering causes that result in gut and digestive diseases. Gut diseases and syndromes may originate from food sensitivities, leaky gut, and other immunity factors, as stated formerly. We will examine the leading causes in more detail, in a later section.

By addressing inflammation, from a more practical perspective, unlike allopathic or alternative treatment options, we can determine the triggering cause of this modern epidemic. We better know the truth before it's too late!

Chapter 8

THE DIABETIC EPIDEMIC

THE SPREAD OF DIABETES AND HOW TO PREVENT IT

Another problem triggered by what we experience daily in our lives e.g eating food also should be stressed and explained in great lengths. The unfavorable issue of diabetes is a long-term metabolic disease in which the system is unable to metabolize and convert carbs, fats and proteins, due to insufficiency or unregulated use of insulin hormone. The are three main kinds of diabetes. They have some symptoms in common and have some complications concerning elevated blood sugar, but they are still different expressions of diabetes.

Diabetes is a disorder in which the system is unable to metabolize and control glucose (blood sugar) and insulin hormone. Glucose is the source that is taken by cells to generate energy. Insulin is the hormone responsible for helping glucose penetrate the cells via cell receptors/pathways. Diabetes symptoms may feature among others tiredness, hunger, thirst, unregulated frequency of urinating, and unexpected weight loss. Extreme blood glucose levels also lead to dizziness, nausea, confusion, and sweating. Diabetes type I is a disorder in which the pancreas can't generate enough levels of insulin to cover the requirements of the system and eventually the blood gets bombarded with excessive sugar levels it is unable to handle. Type II Diabetes is a situation where the cells of the system become sensitive to insulin and can't receive any blood sugar. In Diabetes II, the blood consists of both high levels of sugar and high levels of insulin.

Insulin is a hormone released by the pancreas following the consumption of carb-rich foods like starches, pasta, grains, etc. A regular intake of foods rich in carbs, and specifically white processed sugar, elevates insulin amounts in the blood. Due to the fact that cells do not react properly to insulin and sugar stays in the blood, the pancreas is forced to secrete higher amounts of insulin, in an effort to counteract this sensitivity and resistance. The elevated insulin amounts generate series of unfavorable reactions and disharmony in the system, leading to a wrecked metabolism. Through the regulation of insulin release levels and regulated consumption of carbs, it's possible to regain back the wrecked metabolic function. If this tendency is not inhibited, the pancreas will eventually become worn out and will be unable to generate the required levels necessary for the system to function.

Ever since 2007, it is estimated that in the U.S only, there are over 23 million people suffering from Diabetes. And the sad part is, not all cases are diagnosed or documented. That amounts to 8% of the total U.S population having Diabetes. It also estimated there are around 17.9million diagnosed patients and 5.7 undiagnosed patients. This figure has grown to be double over the years and is constantly on the rise.

The pharmaceutical and medical system concentrates in the regulation of blood sugar and insulin levels using drugs and insulin replacement therapy. But the matter of fact is, if we keep on artificially replacing natural body levels, the system will quit producing amounts of the substance naturally on its own. An organ whose function gets downgraded and is no longer valuable will, as the time passes, become weak and malnourished with decreased power and abilities to function. Therefore, if we replace a compound that the system intends to release itself e.g insulin in this case, the system will eventually be deprived of its ability to secret that compound and will need a replacement.

On the period between 1997 and 2009, the amount of adults affected by Diabetes and taking drugs for their condition has risen 2x, from 5 to 11m (patients taking only drugs), and from 1.1 to 2.9m for those undergoing both drug and insulin replacement therapy. On the contrary, the number of adults taking only insulin has stayed within the same levels (2.3 million patients in total).In the year 2009, 16.3 adult diabetes patients stated getting medication, or insulin, or both whereas 3.2 sufferers stated that they didn't receive any form of pharmaceutical treatment for their diabetes.

The natural healing system advises that we work with our system and not attack it, to clear and recover the impaired organ or body function, while offering all the construction elements needed to release the necessary compounds. So how can we restore the damage caused by such widespread disorder in the Western world? The solution may come off as a surprise to you.

HOW TO INHIBIT DIABETES AND RESTORE BALANCE

The medical community has aimed to treat Diabetes through the prescription of insulin and pills for many years. Doctors though, haven't paid any attention to diet/nutrition and other potential treatment pathways to inhibit the effects of Diabetes or even complete eradicate the disease. What they did though, was to use drugs as the only option to treat such disorder. Still, there are new, fresh and holistic solutions to this issue that have proven to be valuable and victorious.

There was a time when it was acknowledged by the doctor community that diabetes can only be treated but not cured and that insulin and drugs are the only treatment approaches to ease diabetes symptoms. If we pay attention to the average diabetes medicine cabinet, we'll see many different things: pills, syringes, blood test checks/monitors, blood samples, etc. The average price for all these treatment tools is estimated to be a whopping $10K annually (per patient). In the U.S only, millions of people suffer from Diabetes. The disorder has bothered many for ages and we are left wondering, why there is no cure yet or what's the root cause of the issue. Big pharmas are making millions out of people's ill health and suffering, from the prescription drug intake alone.

So how can we change this epidemic and initiate the healing function? As in the case of any natural treatment system, diet is a primary matter. What we choose to ingest clearly influences how good we feel or not. If we address the disorder with only supplements while ignoring our diet choices, we are not making ourselves different from the conventional drug/insulin prescription approach, thinking falsely that we are fixing the issue. This is particularly applicable to scenarios where metabolic function is affected and impaired. The regulation of blood glucose and insulin amounts needs substantial dietary changes. Treating diabetes without any drugs or insulin syringes should be a target and a viable option for anyone affected by the disorder. Common diabetic pills like Actos were labeled with a black warning statement after it was found that they may lead to elevated risk and outburst of bladder cancer in those who took it on regular basis. Actos was also connected to incidents of heart issues and became cancelled in Europe after thousands of patients receiving it experienced heart failures. There is one thing we can tell for sure--this is not a safe pill to take!! You must make the necessary lifestyle and diet adjustment in place of popping potentially dangerous pills.

The American ADA (*American Diabetic Association*) acknowledges the above. Sadly, their diet adjustments aren't reasonable enough when we take a closer look at the nature of the disorder. Why does this happen? The majority of doctors and the medical family in general, do not believe yet that Diabetes regulation is practical and feasible. Sadly, very few people acknowledge efficient treatment of diabetes and this leaves us no other option than to focus on healing diabetes through natural diabetes regulation. Still, it is vital to acknowledge that prior you embark on your natural healing journey, you should bear some things in mind.

Prior following a natural diabetes regulation protocol, discuss the matter with someone that acknowledges and supports natural healing modalities. You have to check that they know any supplements combo, how they work with each other, and if there is possible interference with other substances. Then, start with the following tips and guidelines for efficient natural diabetes regulation:

- You should stay away from foods that are rich in sugar
- Stay away from foat-loaded foods as well. Replace these fattening and unhealthy foods with fruit and veggies portions as they contain fiber and these foods have the potential to decrease blood sugar levels.
- Stay away from foods that contain gluten/white flour and all its byproducts. White, processed flour without fiber make blood sugar levels spike.

- Keep on checking your sugar levels with a blood test monitor. The implementation of natural, drug-free approach doesn't imply that you should throw away all your supplemental tools e.g blood check counters, after taking your first supplement or healthy food.
- Minimize the consumption of red meat in your diet. You can still meet your daily protein intake targets by consuming lean, fat-free cuts, chicken, fatty fish that contains healthy fats like tuna, herring, sardines or salmon, turkey, or rabbit. You can also reap proteins from egg yolks, legumes, and nuts or seeds.
- Limit your salt intake and replace high amounts of salt with aromatic herbs like garlic, ginger, rosemary, or parsley to make your food taste better, minus excess salt. Apart from diet and lifestyle adjustments, there are other healing approaches that yield positive outcomes when it comes to regulating blood sugar and insulin is NOT the solution. In order to receive a diabetes diagnosis, you should be checked for it first. From a doctor's point of view, physiological blood sugar levels should fall between the scale of 70 to 105, while the most appropriate blood sugar levels should be between 85 and 99. Based on ADA guidelines, a blood glucose test between 106 to 126, is considered as "insulin resistance" or "pre-diabetes" condition, and any levels exceeding that mark are considered to be full-blown diabetes.

A test that shows levels below 85 is considered to be hypoglycemia, and a score above 99 is considered to be hyperglycemia. Hypoglycemia is a pathological situation in which the blood glucose levels keep on falling to below normal range levels as a reaction to high carb foods. Hypoglycemia can also occur when one stays too many hours without eating something e.g skipping breakfast.

In case your blood glucose score is under 85, it's is suggested that you eat something every 2-3 hours. You should take a breakfast, snack, lunch, dessert or snack and dinner or even a light snack before sleeping time. There are plenty of healthy snacks to munch on--veggie sticks, fruit, greek yogurt, nuts, seeds, etc. As long as its healthy and nutrient-dense, you can take it.

Now insulin resistance is a condition with elevated blood sugar levels that haven't exceeded yet the max. limit to be considered Diabetes. It's named "pre-diabetes" and is triggered by your cells switching to insulin resistance, preventing glucose to enter the cell and generate energy out of the cell.

A person requires glucose in the body cells to convert it into energy. It is an essential function of your body and life. Both your brain and central nervous system require two elements to survive: fueling source and kick over. Fuel originates from oxygen and sugar molecules. Glucose circulates the blood flow until it gets converted to triglycerides for fat deposition. This is why you should also check your triglyceride levels along with your blood sugar levels. The function of converting glucose into triglycerides requires higher energy levels, leading to a feeling of tiredness after eating something. So when you are following a diet high in carbs and loaded with processed sugar, pasta, pies, white bread, and starches, you won't be able to balance your blood sugar levels.

If you feel lethargic or tired or experience sugar cravings after you eat, this is a sign that you've consumed an excessive amount of carbs. If you feel lethargic and deprived of energy after a meal with little to none carbs, you most likely suffer from insulin resistance.

You should take a healthy breakfast to help improve your hypoglycemia or insulin resistance efforts. As a matter of fact, consuming a breakfast that consists of high quality and good amounts of protein is the only solution to help balance the blood sugar levels in your system. Even if you experience nausea as soon as you wake-up, consuming breakfast is important and taking a breakfast will most likely help improve any symptoms of nausea.

You don't have to swallow the term diabetes for all the symptoms you experience. There is not only one explanation when it comes to deciphering your blood glucose issues. If you've been diagnosed with diabetes, you have to realize that there are some adjustment you can implement to support your condition. Insulin isn't the only path to approach your diagnosis.

As a matter of fact, insulin should not be implemented at all to regulate diabetes type II, because it leads to inflammation, which is unfavorable if you have diabetes. When insulin enters your system (through injection), you are actually exposing yourself to a very high probability of triggering inflammation. There is also a very elevated risk of developing stroke and heart problems. There are other kinds of natural approaches that can accelerate diabetes treatment and regulation. To learn which these approaches are, read on further.

DIABETIC NEUROPATHY AND TREATMENT

Infrared light is considered to be an invisible layer of the general electromagnetic field, which consists of wave patterns that are lengthier than those found in visible red light, but shorter than microwaves or radio waves. The revolutionary discovery of infrared light was initiated by an established astronomer known as Sir William Herschel during the 19th century. While he examined the connection between heat and light, he generated an electromagnetic field through distributing sunlight through a prism form and calculating temperature levels outside the streams of sunlight. This transparent light demonstrated an electromagnetic field with a lower frequency than typical, visible light and longer wave patterns ranging from 0.7 micrometer to 1 micrometer. Following this finding, infrared become considered as a type of invisible light. It became a valuable treatment option and acted as a pain buster for animals and humans alike.

The molecular composition of all living organisms as well as dead organisms is distinguished by its capability to absorb infrared light. This is typically called the "molecular infrared absorption spectrum". Because of its chemical breakdown, infrared light has been successfully applied to the treatment of specific pathological situations. The implementation of infrared light as pain reduction agent emerged in various civilizations and parts across the world, namely by Ancient Greeks, Romans, Egypt, and Asian cultures. A natural administration of herbs and sunlight as a skin treatment agent was also implemented in India, around 1500 BC. Together with the application of natural light, the beaming implementation of man-made light also emerged for the treatment of Tuberculosis. This was initiated by the "father" of up to date light treatment, Neil Finsen. This progress in light treatment in the 20th century, expedited the utilization of synthetic light for the treatment of numerous skin disorders, hair problems, weight control, and faster recovery from painful conditions.

Scientific studies and trials, on the healing impact of infrared light gained ground over the last 40 years. Infrared light healing energy was made suitable for the treatment of numerous skin problems and non-skin problems. Massage experts, physical therapists, doctors and vets have been utilizing infrared light as a healing modality for stomach pain relief, blood flow, headaches, arthritis, sprains, and diabetes ulcers among others. Infrared light has also penetrated the cosmetology/beauty field by combating acne and various other skin disorders or anti-aging applications. Specifically, infrared light acts to fix the destruction of a tissue or cell, by radiating light streams of certain wave patterns. A controlled infrared machine called LED (LIGHT EMITTING DIODE), has been broadly implemented for damage cell rejuvenation all across the globe, with no major side effects. LED devices are available in all kinds of strengths (frequencies and wave patterns) and make an easy to carry and use mobile device for any medical or paramedical expert.

Backed-up scientific evidence has emphasized that diabetes sufferers can be efficiently treated and cured via infrared light therapy. The negative side impact of diabetes triggers numerous medical problems like long-rem muscular pain, poor blood circulation, decrease of balance and loss of sensitivity to stimuli which triggers more life-threatening medical conditions like ulcers and wounds. These medical situations fall under the "Neuropathic Disorders" umbrella. This is triggered by an impair of the nervous system as a result of a direct nerve damage disease like diabetes symptoms or a side impact of a damaging accident or occurrence. The receptors of the nervous system of a diabetic patient may be impaired towards the bad or good side. Some instances of nerve activity loss include numbness, shaking, poor balance/coordination which excess nerve activity triggers pain, tingling sensation, and discomfort in diabetes sufferers.

The medical link between diabetes and infrared light is that the second, offers the light power amount required to kickstart the healing progress. As specified previously, infrared light specific healing is focused on active cells and nerves. In controlled circumstances, infrared light energy is active in human red blood cells, which secrete a cardio-compatible gas (Nitric Oxide), in diabetes sufferers. Infrared light energy amplifies the release of Nitric Oxide gas in cells, which consequently assists in the regulation of blood circulation and cardiovascular function. Diabetic neuropathic diseases keep on being treated through the use of infrared light, by reinstating the vascular and recovery activity of red blood cells.

IRLTT (Infrared Light Therapy Treatment), acts as a suggested cure method for diabetes patients who experience neuropathic diseases. IRLTT morbidly facilitates damaged body balance, numbness in the limbs and sensory nerves by regulating the release of Nitric oxide in blood cells. The treatment course and period varies according to the severity of the neuropathic disease. 8 treatment sessions are required on average (lasting around 30 minutes each), we can experience improvements in type 1 neuropathic diseases and type II diabetes sufferers. The pain reduction facilitated by IRLTT is able to last longer and is a highly sought treatment choice of diabetes patients due to the lack of pills and other pain reduction drugs.

Infrared light also assists in the activation of mitochondria in all living cells. Mitochondria are the power units of blood cells that facilitate cellular development, cellular stability, and cellular boost to carry out certain body tasks. IRLTS responds within mitochondria cells to facilitate pain reduction in diabetic patients.

Infrared light, similar to visible light, consists of numerous color shades with varied frequencies and wave patterns. The application of infrared light on the human skin, gets a varied response as against various wave patterns. The length of absorption can be regulated in regards to the surface exposure of the wound or lesion. For instance, visible light that enters through 10 mm of the skin's depth, needs a wave pattern of 700 nm compared to 1000 nm necessary for organ therapy. Infrared light can enter through depths of 40 mm and is deemed highly efficient in big organ treatment.

Regulating a human's body immune function is more simple with infrared light therapy penetrated through the belly button of the diabetic sufferer. The aortic artery just beneath the belly button after it gets light beams, injects that light through the blood flow and exposed every human cell that it comes in contact with to healing light. In just 20 minutes of light circulation, white blood cells, red blood cells, B-cells, and T-cells are capable of releasing enough oxygen molecules to repair the whole system! Nitric Oxide specifically acts on cellular metabolic function to help the treatment of neuropathic diseases.

Here is an easy formula to better grasp the advantages of infrared light healing:

Evident Light Tissue Treatment Equation:

Visible red light of 700 nm wave pattern enters as deep as 10mm (triggers enough Nitric Oxide). This an efficient healing method for various lesions, infections, wounds, cuts and acupuncture pressure regions.

IRLTS Organ Healing Formula:

Infrared light up to a 1000 nm wave pattern can enter through 40 mm skin depth (enough to release substantial amounts of nitric oxide), capable of treating stomach ulcers, joint impair, bones and deep muscle tissue areas.

The tapping length of infrared light is 4X as much as that of visible light but its therapy outcomes are very efficient in treating organ wounds and deep muscle damage. Diabetes sufferers have to rely on various harsh medical approaches through the rest of their lives. Infrared light therapy for these people gives new hope and makes a great source for efficient recovery as opposed to costly drug usage.

The effective treatment or even cure of every medical situation, has primarily two treatment choices, post-operatively. The first includes prescription of drugs and the second is to facilitate the natural healing process. Infrared light can be used in the second treatment case through its natural stimulation of human cell growth to assist in the healing of important health issues and diabetic neuropathic diseases. All that can be induced without the use of any pills and costly healing options. Therefore, if you are fed up popping pills and look for a natural source to treat your lesions and pains, seek out Infrared Light Treatment.

Infrared Light Therapy has yielded substantial rejuvenation results on diabetic patients and is still a very viable and efficient treatment modality for diabetic sufferers (Diabetes type I and type II). The vibrational infrared light treatment has been shown to raise peripheral sensation in diabetes subjects with diabetic peripheral neuropathy symptoms within only 6 treatment sessions.

Keep in mind that not all the info coming from your doctor's mouth is necessarily accurate or correct. Insulin isn't the only treatment option when it comes to regulating your diabetes. There are numerous independent studies that have shown the healing potential and outcomes of alternative treatment modalities for diabetes. Pills prescribed by doctors, in reality, do more harm than good and lead to inflammation, toxic status, and oxidative damage. You can eradicate this epidemic if you tackle the matter on your own.

It is vital to stay away from drugs as a healing choice. You can be in charge of your own health and still get great outcomes. You may unknowingly mask symptoms by taking drugs, but you may suffer from negative side effects without realizing it at first. Don't fall into the trap that only medication is good for you. If you find the originating cause of the issue and tackle it from the start, this a perfect way to kickstart your recovery journey.

Now, let's examine other connections between cause and outcome. Some stats are really chilling.

Chapter 9

DIABETIC NEUROPATHY

Neuropathy (nerve damage) can be caused by various conditions, ranging from the commonest cause, diabetes, to even treatment regimens like cancer chemotherapy. This condition is sometimes termed peripheral neuropathy, describes multiple health issues involving damage to the peripheral nerves and the symptoms associated with those disorders. Damage to the nerves outside of the central nervous system (brain and spinal cord) causes weakness, altered sensation and numbness in the hands and feet. It may also have an impact on other parts of your body. People usually describe the pain from peripheral neuropathy as sharp, burning, or tingling. Symptoms often get better, particularly when a curable disease causes them. Peripheral neuropathy can be relieved with the use of medications.

Neuropathic pain is a difficult condition to manage. It's a diverse condition that's mostly resistant to widely given painkillers. In a large percentage of patients, current treatment techniques fail to provide adequate or tolerable pain relief. Inadequate diagnosis and a lack of knowledge of the processes involved, poor care of concomitant diseases, wrong understanding or selection of treatment choices, and the use of unsuitable outcomes measurements are the four primary reasons why therapies for neuropathic pain fail.

Causes

Peripheral neuropathy is nerve damage produced by a variety of diseases rather than being a single illness. Peripheral neuropathy can be caused by a myriad of health conditions.

In neuropathy, nerve signaling is interrupted in three ways

- Loss of normal signals
- Sending of inappropriate signals when there is no impulse
- Distortions to the signal being transmitted

Symptoms might range from moderate to severe, although they are seldom fatal. The type of nerve fibers damaged and the type and intensity of injury determine the symptoms. Symptoms might appear for days, weeks, or years. Symptoms may improve on their own in some situations, necessitating no further treatment. Peripheral nerve cells, unlike nerve cells in the central nervous system, continue to develop throughout life.

Only one nerve can be damaged in some types of neuropathy (called mononeuropathy). Multiple mononeuropathy, also known as mononeuropathy multiplex, is a kind of neuropathy that affects two or more nerves in separate anatomical locations. Many, if not all, of the nerves, are damaged (called polyneuropathy).

Diabetes is the commonest cause of PN. There are other common causes such as idiopathic, HIV-related, chemotherapy-related, and autoimmune-related. Autoimmune illnesses are a common cause of peripheral neuropathy. This type of disease in which the immune system attacks itself. Some examples include Sjogren's syndrome, lupus, rheumatoid arthritis, Guillain-Barre syndrome, chronic inflammatory demyelinating polyneuropathy, and vasculitis.

What Role Does Diabetes Play in Causing Neuropathy?

Nerve issues might occur at any time in a person living with diabetes. Neuropathy is sometimes the first indication of diabetes. During the first 10 years after a diabetes diagnosis, significant nerve issues (clinical neuropathy) might occur. The longer the duration a person lives with diabetes, the more likely a neuropathy will develop. Neuropathy affects around half of all diabetics.

Although the specific causes of diabetic neuropathy are unknown, a number of variables may play a role, including:

High blood sugar: High blood glucose damages neurons by causing chemical changes that impede their capacity to send impulses. It can also harm the blood arteries that supply the neurons with oxygen and nourishment. It can also harm the blood arteries that supply the neurons with oxygen and nutrition.

Metabolic factors: High triglyceride and cholesterol levels, in addition to glucose levels, are linked to an increased risk of neuropathy. Neuropathy is more likely to present in people who are overweight or obese.

Genetic Factors: Some hereditary characteristics may predispose some persons to nerve illness more than others.

According to a major American research, 47% of people with diabetes have some form of peripheral neuropathy. At the time of a diabetes diagnosis, neuropathy is predicted to be already present in 7.5% of patients. Distal symmetric polyneuropathy accounts for more than half of all cases. The rest comprises focal syndromes such as carpal tunnel syndrome (14-30%), radiculopathies/plexopathies, and cranial neuropathies. There is a shortage of reliable prevalence statistics for the latter two less frequent disorders.

The absence of standard diagnostic criteria, different ways of choosing patients for research, and different evaluation methodologies all contribute to the vast variation in symmetric diabetic polyneuropathy prevalence data. Furthermore, because many people with the condition are asymptomatic at first, diagnosis relies heavily on a thorough neurologic examination by a primary care physician. Additional diagnostic methods, such as autonomic or quantitative sensory testing, might lead to a greater incidence being documented.

Prevalence of Peripheral Neuropathy in the United States

To acquire a clearer picture of the peripheral neuropathy prevalence in the US, it makes sense to categorize incidence according to cause.

Diabetic neuropathy

The diagnosis of diabetic peripheral neuropathy is based on both clinical indicators and quantitative tests, and it may exist despite the absence of symptoms. Peripheral neuropathy affects 28% of individuals with diabetes in the United States. In a survey of 4400 Belgian patients, researchers discovered that 7.5% already had neuropathy before they were diagnosed with diabetes. After 25 years, the percentage of people with neuropathy had risen to 45%. Diabetic neuropathy is prevalent among the hospital clinic population in the United Kingdom, with a frequency of about 29%.

Diabetic peripheral neuropathy can have profound implications. Diabetes mellitus significantly increases the risk of lower limb amputation, with around 50% of diabetics developing a foot ulcer over their lifespan. Furthermore, neuropathic pain and reduced sensation can lead to various negative consequences, including falls, lower quality of life, limitations in daily activities, and symptoms of depression.

HIV-associated sensory peripheral neuropathy

The most frequent neurological consequence of HIV infection is peripheral neuropathy. Despite this, it is underdiagnosed and undertreated. This illness, which has a detrimental influence on HIV/AIDS patients' quality of life, comes in various clinical forms, including HIV-associated. The most prevalent kind of HIV neuropathy is sensory neuropathy (HIV-SN), which affects up to two-thirds of individuals with advanced illness in some situations.

Primary HIV-associated distal sensory polyneuropathy (HIV-DSP) and ART toxic neuropathy (ATN) are the two main forms of HIV-associated distal sensory peripheral neuropathies that afflict 30–67% of individuals with advanced HIV.

Postherpetic Neuralgia

PHN is a form of NP caused by the reactivation of the herpes zoster virus. The virus persists in an inactive state within the sensory ganglion of the spinal cord until the patient's immunocompetence deteriorates due to aging, HIV infection, cancer, or immunosuppressive treatment, at which point it can reactivate.

According to data from *Clinical Infectious Diseases,* the total incidence rate of PHN was 57.5 cases per 100,000 person-years (95 percent confidence interval: 56.0-59.0). Researchers also discovered that the proportion of people with HZ who acquired PHN increased from 2007 to 2018 compared to 1994 to 2006.

Chemotherapy-induced peripheral neuropathy

This is the most prevalent complication of neurological cancer therapy. It is a chemotherapy-related side effect that is dose-dependent. The sensory nerves in the posterior ganglion of the spinal cord are damaged by these drugs. The pain and numbness in patients with CIPN are described as symmetric and distal, with a "glove and stocking" distribution. Approximately one-third of cancer patients are given chemotherapy. The majority of individuals get neuropathic symptoms within six months after starting chemotherapy. As the treatment continues, the symptoms may increase. In many situations, once the therapy is stopped, it improves.

Guillain-Barre Syndrome (GBS)

Guillain-Barre syndrome (GBS) has been studied in over 30 population studies inthe past 5 decades, most of which have shown a yearly prevalence in the range of 10 to 20 per 100,000 population. The condition appears evenly distributed throughout the world, and incidence rates are probably fairly stable over time. The annual prevalence seemed to rise from 1-2 per 100 000 in 1953-6 to 2-7 per 100,000 in 1970-80 in Olmsted county, Rochester, USA.

Although GBS incidence is low (although not very low, since it is roughly half that of multiple sclerosis), the cumulative effect of life-long impairment in young people constitutes a significant but underappreciated public health issue. After a year, 13% of 79 patients in a recent population-based survey in southeast England need assistance to walk, a handicap that is likely to be permanent. The illness can strike anyone at any age, from infancy to old life. There is a more or less linear increase in incidence with age, which is consistent with a decrease in immune suppressor systems as people become older and, as a result, an increased vulnerability to autoimmune illness.

Chronic Inflammatory Demyelinating Polyradiculoneuropathy (CIDP)

CIDP (classified as an acquired idiopathic demyelinating neuropathy with a progressive phase > eight weeks) has relatively limited epidemiological data, in contrast to GBS. It's definitely a rare illness, but the neurophysiological and nerve biopsy tests needed to detect it are complex. Thus, it's likely underdiagnosed. There are currently no accurate population estimates of its prevalence. However, some data shows a frequency of at least 1 per 100 000 people.

Carpal tunnel syndrome

This condition occurs as a result of median nerve compression as it travels through the wrist's transverse carpal ligament. It is a prevalent diagnosis in outpatient neurology and rheumatology clinics, but there is surprisingly little information regarding its prevalence in the general population.

In a study, researchers identified carpal tunnel syndrome in 3-4% of the women and was present, though undiagnosed, in the other 5.8%. Men, on the other hand, had a prevalence rate of just 0-6 percent. The female to male ratio in age-adjusted sex-specific rates was 3:1. Men's rates rose with age, whereas women's rates peaked in the 45 to 54 age period.

There are several risk factors for developing carpal tunnel syndrome. In retrospective investigations of clinic-based case series, associations with diabetes, hypothyroidism, rheumatoid arthritis, amyloidosis, pregnancy, and hemodialysis have been discovered. The majority of pregnancy-related problems go away on their own once the baby is born.

Alcohol

People who abuse alcohol are more likely to develop peripheral nerve damage. The question of whether this is due to a direct toxic impact of alcohol or a chronic nutritional deficit has been debated for a long time. In the United States, it is believed that 25% to 66% of chronic alcoholics suffer from neuropathy; however, the real prevalence in the general population is unclear. The bulk of the patients were middle-class working males, and those who drank continuously were more impacted than those who drank episodically.

Traditional Avenues Associated with the Treatment of Neuropathy

There are a variety of therapies available to assist in alleviating symptoms and peripheral neuropathy. The phrase "traditional/conventional neuropathy therapy" refers to treatment methods that doctors have given for a long time. These therapy approaches are backed by science and have a track record of success. The type of treatment for peripheral neuropathy is determined by the etiology. Physical therapy, surgery, and injections for increased nerve pressure are some of the most frequent therapies. Approaches can be pharmacological and non-pharmacological

Medical Treatment

Over-the-counter non-steroidal anti-inflammatory medicines like ibuprofen and aspirin are examples of this regimen. Headaches, stomach discomfort, stomach ulcers, dizziness, and elevated blood pressure are all possible side effects. These medicines can assist with pain, but they may not be enough. More potent medications, such as antidepressants or anticonvulsants, may be administered as a result, and they are often more successful. In fact, research supports the use of older antidepressant drugs to treat neuropathy. Newer medicines are usually more successful.

Clomipramine and Amitriptyline, on the other hand, have been proven to function better for neuropathy than the newer Serotonin Reuptake Inhibitors in this study (SSRIs). While SSRIs are more successful in treating depression, they have less of an effect on neuropathy. Prozac, Zoloft, Cymbalta, Celexa, and Nardil are some of the most well-known brands. Dry mouth, headaches, and sexual dysfunction are all common adverse effects.

Anticonvulsants are also useful in the treatment of neuropathy pain, although there isn't enough evidence to back them up. However, patients using these drugs, which include Gabapentin and Tiagabine, have experienced less discomfort. This implies that, while studies may not reveal why they function, they appear to do so. Gralise, Neuraptine, and Lyrica are brand names of the most often prescribed anticonvulsants. Dizziness, tiredness, nausea, sleepiness, and weight gain are some of the side effects.

Narcotic medications reduce neuronal excitability (which causes pain) by binding to specific receptors in the brain and peripheral nervous system. Short-acting or long-acting opioid pain medications are available. Codeine, hydrocodone, morphine, and oxycodone are common examples. Nausea, vomiting, and constipation are common adverse effects.

Surgical Treatment

For some kinds of neuropathies, surgery is the preferred therapy. Nerve roots that are compressed by protruding disks ("pinched nerves") in the back or neck are often treated surgically to release the afflicted nerve root and allow it to recover. Neurosurgical decompression is frequently used to treat facial trigeminal neuralgia. A single nerve injury (mononeuropathy) caused by compression, trapping, or, in rare cases, tumors or infections, may necessitate surgery to relieve the nerve compression. Surgical surgery does not assist polyneuropathies with more widespread nerve degeneration, such as diabetic neuropathy.

Surgery or interventional treatments that seek to relieve pain by cutting or damaging nerves are usually ineffective because they exacerbate nerve injury, and the portions of the peripheral and central nervous systems above the incision frequently keep sending pain signals ("phantom pain"). These surgeries have mostly been superseded by more advanced and less harmful treatments such as electrically stimulating remaining peripheral nerve fibers or pain-processing regions of the spinal cord or brain.

Other Approaches to Treatment of Neuropathy

Low-Intensity Red Light

The Semmes-Weinstein 10-g monofilament is commonly used to diagnose diabetic peripheral neuropathy (SWM). Recent research suggests that treating diabetic individuals with monochromatic near infrared red energy (MIRE) can temporarily improve their foot sensitivity to the SWM. In individuals with diabetic peripheral neuropathy, pulsed infrared light treatment (PILT) has been proven to improve peripheral sensitivity. However, most trials are short-term, with individuals getting just 6–20 treatment sessions.

Vibration Therapy

Whole-Body Vibration (WBV) training is a novel form of somatosensory stimulation (SSS) exercise that has gained popularity in sports training and rehabilitation over the past ten years. WBV improves physical strength and balance with time. The treatment modality was shown in a recent study to have an influence on the pain level of a diabetic patient with neuropathy.

Although peripheral neuropathy is thought to be progressive and permanent, the patient's (Michigan Diabetic Neuropathy Score) MDNS score decreased considerably during the WBV trials. Though research is still in its early phases, combining WBV with other therapeutic treatment methods might be beneficial.

Nutrition

People with diabetic neuropathy should try to maintain the blood glucose levels recommended by their doctors. To do these, they need to avoid processed carbohydrates such as sweets, sugary beverages, etc. Instead, focus on portion control and carbohydrates derived from high-fiber/whole grains. Vegetables, fruits, low- or nonfat dairy, and lean meats are also excellent sources of energy and nourishment. These dietary precautions may not cure current nerve damage, but they will help you avoid additional injury.

Alternative medicine's claims pique the interest of many individuals. It sounds easy to add a supplement to food tea in order to get rid of the constant pain. While there is some validity to a number of these supplements, the majority of alternative medicine options possess little to no scientific backing, and many have no observable effects superior to placebo. This effect occurs because you already have faith in the efficacy of the tea or supplement and this plays a psychological trick on you that reduces your sensitivity to pain.

Of course, taking vitamins and supplements is beneficial for your body as a whole. However, if you're not having enough of these substances in your diet, taking extra supplements isn't likely to treat your neuropathy. Taking additional supplements, on the other hand, is unlikely to help treat neuropathy if a patient isn't receiving enough of these nutrients in their diet. That's because everything the body doesn't require to function will be flushed away. There's also the danger of overdoing it. Taking excessive quantities of some vitamins like A and E is detrimental to health.

Exercise and Lifestyle Changes

Although many of the most frequent causes of peripheral neuropathy are incurable, it's essential to recognize that regular exercise can not only help avoid some of them but it's also been shown to help relieve some of the condition's most unpleasant symptoms. The major treatment method for type 2 diabetes patients is aerobic exercise. In addition to endurance training, diabetes type 2 patients are given segmental strength training of the primary muscle groups.

Other lifestyle modification strategies include proper foot care e.g by wearing well-fitted, padded shoes and minimizing pressure to areas like knees and elbow. These measures help to reduce pain and the risk of trauma. Smoking can obstruct blood flow and cause blood vessels to constrict. Cessation of smoking improves blood flow, and blood vessels become healthier. Massages and acupuncture are examples of might help patients relax and feel better. Essential oils, like chamomile and lavender, can assist in relieving pain and increasing blood flow throughout the body.

Spinal Cord Stimulation (SCS)

SCS is a type of pain neuromodulation. A fully implanted SCS system consists of two parts: electrodes (or leads) and an implantable pulse generator (IPG). SCS modifies local neurochemistry in dorsal horns by implanted electrodes, reducing the hyperexcitability of neurons with variable pulse-width modulation. In two open-label controlled studies, adjuvant SCS for the treatment of refractory painful diabetic peripheral neuropathy showed a substantial decrease in pain intensity ratings that lasted at least six months.

Transcutaneous Electrical Nerve Stimulation (TENS)

It is a non-invasive pain treatment technique that may be utilized for a variety of ailments. The treatment involves placing electrodes to the skin at the location of pain or near related nerves and then providing a mild electrical current. TENS has been demonstrated to alleviate neuropathic symptoms linked with diabetes in several studies, despite the lack of data from controlled clinical trials to generally confirm its efficacy for peripheral neuropathies.

Experiences of People Seeking Care for Neuropathy

The primary symptoms of peripheral neuropathy are neuromuscular, with physical pain in the feet, hands, arms, back, and knees. Numbness and tingling, being the most common complaints. Furthermore, comorbid disorders, such as depression, are typical consequences of chronic pain, and they contribute to patients' everyday impairment and disability. Despite variations in the presentation of their symptoms, investigators discovered that individuals with the disease had comparable treatment and care routes, according to a study of persons living with the ailment.

Clinic administrative difficulties lead to patients with peripheral neuropathy receiving less-than-optimal treatment. Because the situation is not considered an emergency, the already overburdened personnel are unable to respond quickly and comprehensively. Even while the number of dedicated pain clinics is growing across the world, only a tiny percentage of patients are referred to pain experts. According to the findings of a UK research of 703 individuals with neuropathic pain, the majority (79%) had been in pain for more than a year before receiving a referral to a pain clinic. This delay has a negative impact on their clinical care and long-term results.

However, a substantial number of patients will receive effective pain reduction and improved quality of life with adequate treatment. Unfortunately, evidence suggests that therapeutic treatment of neuropathic pain is frequently insufficient. An explanation for this is that pain perception is influenced by three aspects: psychological, psychobehavioral, and sociocultural factors. Many neuropathy patients say their pain has affected their emotions, sleep, relationships, and ability to operate. This discovery is comparable to that of Hensing et al. in 2007, who demonstrated cases of exaggerated pain and chronic pain repercussions in neuropathic patients, where contact with a nightdress generated a considerable stimulus that would be insignificant in a healthy patient.

Though combination treatment is superior to administering a single pharmacological agent, it may not be enough to relieve pain completely. Non-pharmaceutical therapies, such as physiotherapy, counseling, or alternative approaches, may also be necessary. According to specific research, cognitive behavioral therapy can help people with chronic pain reduce discomfort and improve positive behavior expression, evaluation, and coping. Relaxation treatments such as progressive muscle relaxation, regulated breathing, guided visualization, and hypnosis are also beneficial.

References

1. Pop-Busui R, Boulton AJ, Feldman EL, Bril V, Freeman R, Malik RA, et al. Diabetic Neuropathy: A Position Statement by the American Diabetes Association. *Diabetes Care*. 2017;40(1):136–154.10.2337/dc16-2042.

2. Gregg EW, Gu Q, Williams D, de Rekeneire N, Cheng YJ, Geiss L, et al. Prevalence of lower extremity diseases associated with normal glucose levels, impaired fasting glucose, and diabetes among U.S. adults aged 40 or older. *Diabetes Res Clin Pract*. 2007;77(3):485–488.10.1016/j.diabres.2007.01.005.

3. Tesfaye S, Stevens LK, Stephenson JM, Fuller JH, Plater M, Ionescu-Tirgoviste C, et al. Prevalence of diabetic peripheral neuropathy and its relation to glycaemic control and potential risk factors: the EURODIAB IDDM Complications Study. *Diabetologia*. 1996;39(11):1377–1384

4. Abbott CA, Malik RA, van Ross ER, Kulkarni J, Boulton AJ. Prevalence and characteristics of painful diabetic neuropathy in a large community-based diabetic population in the U.K. *Diabetes Care*. 2011;34(10):2220–2224.10.2337/dc11-1108

5. Arya Shah et. al. Incidence and disease burden of chemotherapy-induced peripheral neuropathy in a population-based

cohort. *J Neurol Neurosurg Psychiatry.* 2018 Jun; 89(6): 636–641. 10.1136/jnnp-2017-317215

6. Cabezas-Cerrato J The prevalence of clinical diabetic poly-neuropathy in Spain: a study in primary care and hospital clinic groups. Neuropathy Spanish Study Group of the Spanish Diabetes Society (SDS). *Diabetologia.* 1998;41(11):1263–1269

7. Cozolino L.J. *The Neuroscience of Psychotherapy: Building and Rebuilding the Human Brain.* 1st ed. W.W. Norton & Company Inc.; New York, NY, USA: 2002. pp. 13–30.

8. Linden D.E. How psychotherapy changes the brain-The contribution of functional neuroimaging. *Mol. Psychiatry.* 2006;11:528–538. doi: 10.1038/sj.mp.4001816.

9. Slangen R, Schaper NC, Faber CG, Joosten EA, Dirksen CD, van Dongen RT, et al. Spinal cord stimulation and pain relief in painful diabetic peripheral neuropathy: a prospective two-center randomized controlled trial. Diabetes Care. 2014;37(11):3016–24.

10. De Vos CC, Meier K, Zaalberg PB, Nijhuis HJ, Duyvendak W, Vesper J, et al. Spinal cord stimulation in patients with painful diabetic neuropathy: a multicenter randomized clinical trial. Pain. 2014;155(11):2426–31.

11. Hong J. Whole Body Vibration Therapy for Diabetic Peripheral Neuropathic Pain: A Case Report. *Health Science Journal* 2011;5(1):66-71.

12. Front Cell Neurosci. 2014; 8: 102.

13. John L. Dobson, Jim McMillan, and Li Li Benefits of exercise intervention in reducing neuropathic pain. *Front Cell Neurosci* 2014 doi: 10.3389/fncel.2014.00102

14. MIRE Mark W. Powell, MD; Dale E. Carnegie, DPM; and Thomas J. Burke, PhD. Reversal of Diabetic Peripheral Neuropathy and New Wound Incidence: The Role of MRE. *Adv Skin Wound Care* 2004;17:295-6, 298-300.

15. https://www.ninds.nih.gov/Disorders/Patient-Caregiver-Education/Fact-Sheets/Peripheral-Neuropathy-Fact-Sheet

16. Hurley R, Adams M & Benzon H. Neuropathic pain: treatment guidelines and updates. *Curr Opin Anaesthesiol* 2013;26(5):580–587.

17. Hensing G.K.E., Sverker A.M., Leijon G.S. Experienced dilemmas of everyday life in chronic neuropathic pain patients-Results from a critical incident study. *Scand. J. Caring Sci.* 2007;21:147–154. doi: 10.1111/j.1471-6712.2007.00450.x.

Chapter 10

THE NEGATIVE EFFECTS OF
SUGAR ON NEUROPATHY

S ugar is found naturally in every food in which carbohydrate is present; foods like fruits, grains, dairy (lactose), and vegetables (Fructose) have natural sugar present in them. When you eat whole foods with raw sugar, there is little or no damage that can occur; high Consumption of these foods reduces the risks of chronic heart disease, diabetes, high blood pressure, and even some Cancer. However, when an individual consumes the sugar in excess, it causes significant threats to the health of such individual.

Insulin is a natural hormone synthesized by the pancreas that regulates how the body uses and stores sugar; when excess sugar is consumed excessively, the presence of insulin is doubled in the bloodstream, this makes the walls of the arteries get inflamed, they grow thicker than they ought to be and more inflexible, this increases the workload of the heart, causing diseases like stroke, heart attack, heart failure and damage to nerves.

Diabetes happens when the body finds it difficult to effectively and efficiently regulate the amount of sugar in the blood. Neuropathy is any ailment or disease that occurs as a result of damage to the peripheral nervous system. Diabetic neuropathy occurs when the peripheral nervous system of an individual has been compromised and begins to malfunction as a result of excess sugar intake. Diabetic neuropathy is a common complication of type 1 and types two diabetes; It occurs when the sugar present in the blood remains high for an extended period without adequate treatment by a doctor. This complication develops slowly and gradually, most times over a decade. Complications resulting from diabetic neuropathy include; Numbness and discomfort in your feet and hands, muscle wasting, bloating, constipation, excessive or decreased sweating. There are various kinds of diabetic neuropathy that affect different areas of your body.

ROLES SUGAR PLAYS IN CAUSING DIABETES

Recently the United Nations stated that for the very first time in human history, chronic non-communicable sicknesses such as cancer, diabetes, and heart disease had more significant threats to our health worldwide than infectious diseases. The attention of most researchers was on alcohol, tobacco; some researchers even focused more on obesity. Still, in 2011 it was discovered that over the past 50 years, Consumption of sugar had increased worldwide, so researchers began to turn their attention towards sugar. It was found that excess sugar intake is one of the leading causes of so many complicated health conditions in the world.

Sugar can occur naturally in certain foods, as stated earlier in this chapter; it is also essential to know that sugar can also be added to food and drink by food manufacturing companies or by us in our homes to make them sweet. These added sugars are also called 'free sugars'. Table sugars that we add to our cereals, caster sugar used in baking, sugars in ready meals, cakes, soda drinks, smoothies, syrups, honey, and even pure fruit juices are examples of 'free sugar'. It is essential to know that sucrose or table sugar is mainly referred to as sugar. Sucrose is made up of glucose and Fructose. When sucrose is consumed, the glucose and Fructose present in it are separated in your small intestine before they become absorbed into your bloodstream; this causes an increase in sugar levels in your blood and causes the pancreas to release insulin. Insulin acts to transport glucose from the bloodstream to cells in your body, where it can be metabolized to provide energy for usage.

On the other hand, Fructose is majorly carried to your liver, where it is metabolized to glucose to provide energy or converted to fat for storage. Now, when excess sugar is consumed, insulin carries excess glucose to cells; after the cells have metabolized this glucose into energy needed, the excess remains are converted into fatty acids and stored as fat. Fructose present in the liver under normal conditions will be converted to fat for storage. Still, in diabetes, where the Fructose is in excess, it elevates triglycerides levels, leading to an increase in the risk of heart disease, gout, and fatty liver. Studies have shown that individuals who frequently drink sugar-sweetened beverages or drinks have a 25% risk of type 2 diabetes. Significant research has also shown that drinking one sugar-sweetened glass per day increases your risk by 13%, independent of any increase in weight. It results in. nations where sugar is highly consumed, have the highest rates of type 2 diabetes. The excessive intake of sugar increases diabetes both directly and indirectly. It directly increases the risk because of the effect of Fructose on your livers which are; enhancing fatty liver, inflammation, and localized insulin resistance; these could lead to abnormal production of insulin by the pancreas and increase the risk of type 2 diabetes. Indirectly, it increases the risk of diabetes by adding weight and increased fat in the body, which are independent risk factors of diabetes. Studies have shown that abnormal sugar intake disrupts the signalling of a hormone that promotes feelings of fullness, resulting in overeating and unnecessary weight gain; this hormone is known as Leptin. It is essential to understand that natural sugars don't have the same effect as this 'free sugar'.

According to the statistics report, crude estimates showed that in the US as of 2018, 34.2million people of all ages, or 10.5% of the US population, had diabetes. 34.1 million Adults, people aged 18 years or older, or 13.0% of all US adults, had diabetes, and 1 in 5 of them doesn't know they have it. Studies have shown that in the United States of America, diabetes is the seventh leading cause of death. Diabetes is the number 1 leading cause of kidney failure, lower-limb amputations, and loss of sight in adults. According to World Health Organization (WHO), 422 million people worldwide have diabetes, especially in low- and middle-income countries, and diabetes is one of the leading causes of death worldwide. Diabetes is the only condition in the United States that continues to inflict, and there is a massive increase in the number of people it imposes. As of today, over 30 million Americans live and from this life-threatening condition.

RELATIONSHIP BETWEEN OBESITY AND DIABETES

There is a close relationship between type 2 diabetes and obesity; it is essential to know that being overweight or obese increases the risk of having diabetes. One of the direct impacts of excess sugar in the blood is that excess glucose and Fructose that remain after metabolizing to produce energy are converted to fat for storage; accumulation of these fats leads to diabetes, type 2 in particular. When an individual has an abnormally high Body Mass Index(BMI), fat cells release chemicals that promote inflammation; these chemicals make the body less sensitive to insulin by interrupting insulin cells responsible for a response, making it challenging to respond to insulin activities. Obesity also triggers adipocytes to produce high quantities of fatty acids, hormones, pro-inflammatory cytokines, and some other factors that promote insulin resistance in the body. When accompanied by malfunctioning pancreatic Islet beta-cells (the cells responsible for releasing insulin), this insulin resistance leads to the inability or failure of the body to control blood glucose levels. It is also essential that of the two types of diabetes, obesity is mainly associated with type 2. Studies have shown that in the United States of America, the obesity prevalence was about 42.4% in 2017-2018. The research was done, and it was discovered that from 1999-2000 through 2017-2018, the prevalence of obesity increased from 30.5% to 42.4%. During the same time, it was also discovered that the most severe obesity increased from 4.7% to 9.2%. These, among many other factors, are the leading cause of the increase in diabetes in the United States. Over the past 25 years, scientists have seen a sporadic rise in obesity across Africa. In the past 25 years, in Egypt, the percentage of obese people has increased from 34% to 39% and 8% to 22% in Ghana. In England, research was done, and it was discovered that in 2019, 28% of the population in England were obese. Taking a close look at these countries mentioned, you would see why many people in the United States are at a high risk of getting diabetes.

Obesity is one of the leading causes of death in the United States of America; the United States, according to the most recent study done by the World Health Organization (WHO), is the 12th country with the highest number of Obese people in the world, with 36.2% of the population being obese. Many questions have been asked, and people have come up with various answers as to what could be the cause of the recent obesity epidemic in the united states. The US department of agriculture reported that the average American consumed close to 20% more calories in the year 2000 than they did in 1983; this is because there has been a boom in meat consumption among the American populace. Consumption of added fats also increased to almost two-thirds over the same length of time, and Consumption of grain increased approximately 45% since 1970. The reason for this recent increase in obesity, according to research published by World Health Organization (WHO), is what we eat, not how much we eat. There has been an increase in fast food consumption, which has contributed significantly to obesity in the United States; fast food makes up 11% of the average American diet. Diet is greatly mistaken for nutrition; companies send consumers mixed messages as processed food, and drive-thru meals are branded as fast, filling delicious and cheap food. In the 1990s, Companies began to manipulate data to confuse consumers. The population at large, low-fat and fat-free goods were no longer in the market and supermarkets. They blamed the reason for the increase in obesity on fat rather than on sugar decades after, and we still find it challenging to believe products that are fat-free and full-flavoured. People are now compelled to blame the Consumption of red meat, wheat, fat, and sugar for being fat when we know the problem is straightforward.

COMPLICATIONS ASSOCIATED WITH OBESITY EXCEPT FOR DIABETES

Obesity is a complex health issue responsible for many life-threatening diseases except diabetes, resulting from behaviour, and sometimes it could be hereditary. Conditions like Cushing's disease and polycystic ovary syndrome cause obesity. Steroids and anti-depressants can also cause weight gain. Obese or overweight individuals are at higher risk for various illnesses and health conditions. Obesity is responsible for diseases like hypertension (high blood pressure), stroke, gall bladder disease, osteoarthritis(a degradation of cartilage and bone within a joint), coronary heart disease, breathing problems, sleep apnea, various kinds of cancer, high LDL cholesterol, low HDL cholesterol and high levels of triglycerides(dyslipidemia). Obesity also has adverse effects on the psychological health of individuals. Mental illnesses like depression, anxiety, obsessive-compulsive disorder, eating disorder, personality disorder, low self-esteem, and so many other mental disorders.

CONSEQUENCES OF EXCESS SUGAR IN THE BRAIN

The brain, a perfectly tuned organ, makes use of the highest amount of energy in the body than any other part of the body, and glucose is its primary source of energy, The effect of diabetes on the brain is rarely spoken about; it is highly imperative to understand that because glucose is the brain's primary source of energy, excess intake of sugar will have significant adverse effects on the brain. There's inflammation in both large and tiny blood vessels. As a result, insufficient nutrient reaches the brain. Diabetes consequences on the brain are not present immediately.

Excess sugar consumption impedes the cognitive skills and self-control of an individual. Excess Consumption of sweet food produces addiction-like effects in the brain leading to the loss of self-control, abnormal weight gain, and overeating. Foods rich in sugar help enhance regions of the brain responsible for reward response and promote a heightened feeling of hunger compared to those relatively low in sugar. Recent studies have shown that sugar can be more addictive than cocaine. A slight increase in the average sugar level of the body could have significant impacts on the brain. Excess sugar intake causes inflammation in the brain, leading to difficulties in memory. Also, the ability to process emotions is reduced in patients with diabetes. Problems in learning, memory, motor sped, deterioration of mental capacity, and other cognitive functions. Damage to tiny blood vessels present in the brain affects the brain's white matter, a part of the brain where nerves communicate with themselves. This could result in vascular dementia. Effects of diabetes on the brain are common in the two types of diabetes (type 1 and type 2), although they are prominent in patients with type 2. By regulating diabetes through adequate treatment and changes in lifestyle, the effects of diabetes on the brain can be controlled. Inadequate sugar in the body can also have adverse effects on the brain.

EFFECTS OF EXCESS SUGAR ON THE IMMUNE SYSTEM

In the presence of excess sugar in the body, the body becomes susceptible to several kinds of disease; the body becomes weak in fighting against toxic substances like bacteria and viruses because the immune system has been compromised. Recent studies have shown that an increase in sugar consumption suppresses or weakens the immune system. Frequent intake of food rich in sugar reduces the body's ability to fight off diseases. White blood cells are also known as 'killer cells', are weakened by excess calories in the blood. A study was carried out, and it was discovered that monocytes, a certain kind of leucocytes (white blood cells), become inflamed when cultured in Fructose. It is also known that dendritic cells (antigen-presenting cells), also called accessory cells and are very important in the immune system, become inflamed when exposed to excess Fructose. When these cells are compromised, the body's ability to ward off disease reduces. What is essential to understand is that sugar contains so many calories and excess calories in the blood affect the immune, nervous system negatively.

EFFECTS OF EXCESS SUGAR ON LIFE SPAN

Just like every other disease, diabetes affects the life span depending on how early it was diagnosed, the complications present, and the presence of preexisting conditions, irrespective of what type of diabetes is considered. Key statistics on diabetes show that individuals with type 2 diabetes have their life span shortened by ten years. Individuals with type 1 have a shorter life. Their life span is reduced by 20 years. Individuals with type 1 diabetes develop diabetes at a very young age compared to those with type 2. As a result, they spend a more extended period living with the disease. Improvements and upgrades in the medical treatment of diabetes have provided ways in which the life span of a diabetic patient could be significantly longer. After a particular period, unusually high blood sugar makes the body susceptible to various complications, such as diabetic retinopathy, cardiovascular disease, kidney disease, increased blood pressure, and high cholesterol. Significant damage is done to some vital organs of the body, reducing the efficiency of these organs and ultimately reduces the life span.

The centres for disease control and prevention (CDC) did a study and discovered that 24% of the 30.3 million people who have diabetes in the United States were diagnosed late. Sometimes diabetes is misdiagnosed; diabetes is a condition that can result in life-long disabilities. Few cases can lead to a date, so when treatment is delayed, these risks are increased. In a weak attempt by medical doctors to manage the disease, diabetes gets complicated and more profound; the patients eventually have to use the more expensive services of the hospital to make more money for them. There are so many complications associated with misdiagnosis or late diagnosis of diabetes. A recent study released by diabetes United kingdom revealed 7,370 amputations in a year are carried out because of diabetes; it was also revealed that 80% of these amputations were avoidable. Still, due to the negligence of the doctor, it had to happen. These amputations mostly begin as treatable foot infections. Still, the doctors want the patient to use the more sophisticated services of the hospital, so they keep them in the hospital and make little or no efforts to care for the individual, the infections spread across the foot into the leg and ultimately leads to amputation.

Blindness is another severe complication of misdiagnosed or late diagnosis of diabetes. Diabetic retinopathy disrupts the blood vessels present in the light-sensitive tissue that lines the back of the eye, called the retina. Controlling or adequate care for patients with diabetes can delay vision loss, but diabetes retinopathy often goes unnoticed until patients become blind. Damage to blood vessels in the kidney (diabetic neuropathy, making its work less efficient, is another complication. Urinary tract infections, strokes, heart attacks, and degeneration of the nerves (diabetic neuropathy) are also complications resulting from misdiagnosis and late diagnosis.

Diabetes imposes a significant amount of burden on society in the form of medicals costs, loss in productivity, intangible expenses, reduced quality of living, and premature mortality. According to a study, the total calculated cost of diagnosed diabetes in 2017, according to a survey, is $327 billion, $237 billion in direct medical expenses, and $90 billion in reduced productivity inclusive.

Asides from going to the hospital for medical check-up, there are various ways that individuals with diabetes can care for themselves without having to spend too much. Organize a diabetes meal plan, get help from your doctor, consume lower calories, sugar, saturated fat, trans- fat, and salt, and eat meals like whole grain, bread, crackers, rice, or pasta. Fruits and vegetables drink water instead of regular soda. Stress also increases the blood sugar in diabetes, so avoid stress and exercise regularly. Irrespective of how good you feel, make sure you take your drugs regularly until the doctor says you are done with the medication and avoid smoking, excessive drinking of alcohol because these things can lead to complications in diabetes. Check your blood pressure regularly. The extent to which an individual can care for one-self is highly dependent on the stage of diabetes; that's why early di-agnosis is essential.

Chapter 11

STATINS AND NEUROPATHY

The pharmaceutical industry has never been entirely immune to controversy. In 2019, Gallaghar highlighted the fair uproar surrounding an exponential prescription of statins and their side effects. Around 74.3 million people in the UK alone are on statin therapy. These include UK's former health minister, Lib Dem, who was prescribed statins after a cardiac stroke in 2018. Lib joined voice with the group of already skeptical scientists headed by Dr. Aseem Malhotra (1). Dr. Malhotra, serving as a cardiologist in the NHS and other signatories, complained about the lack of transparency and quoted many patients who discontinued statins, shifted to a low-fat vegan diet, and experienced the side-effects to disappear temporarily. They called for a parliamentary inquiry into the statin controversy (2). Similar concerns were highlighted in the US and the world over. The question, however, remains; Are the fear of cholesterol and increased statin prescription or propagation of the multi-billion-dollar, anti-cholesterol, and low-fat diet industry, justified?

1. What are statins?

Statins, or HMG-CoA reductase inhibitors, are cholesterol-lowering drugs that are prescribed to patients with a history of or at risk of cardiovascular complications (3). They have pleiotropic and antiatherosclerotic effects due to their cholesterol-lowering (hypolipidemic) properties. They mainly function by affecting the cholesterol synthesis pathways in the human body. Statins also affect other metabolic processes and enzymes in the mitochondria that are responsible for producing the energy needed by the skeletal muscles to function and peripheral nervous system to send and receive messages or neural impulses (4, 5, 6).

2. Why are they prescribed?

The primary reason for prescribing statins is to lower cholesterol. Cholesterol could accumulate in the body due to many different reasons such as diabetes, obesity and foreseeable cardiovascular complications such as coronary heart disease, heart attack, and heart failure. People with diabetes are, therefore, prescribed statins because they are believed to be at a greater risk of atherosclerotic cardiovascular disease but risk chances for new-onset diabetes (NOD) (3). Researchers reiterate that statins create a substantial risk for new-onset diabetes, but there is yet no consensus on the exact molecular mechanism (4).

About pancreatic beta cells, responsible for the production of insulin and glucose metabolism, the statins alter insulin secretion, working of the Ca^{2+} gated channels, or induce oxidative stress. Other metabolic alterations include those of adipocyte differentiation mechanisms, in which case the preadipocytes are incapable of producing glucose sensitizing hormone or mature adipocytes secrete adiponectin, which is known to cause insulin resistance (4). Other anomalies include genetic or epigenetic predisposition (5).

The most widely accepted mechanism to induce new-onset diabetes is the ability of statins to reduce insulin secretion and sensitivity to insulin (6). It is important to note that because patients with familial hypercholesterolemia have a mutated low-density lipoprotein receptor or LDLR gene, they have protection against developing type 2 diabetes (7). It does not appeal to logic, therefore, to continue prescribing these drugs to diabetic patients only as a prevention against future cardiac complications. An extensive study conducted on 1.9 million diabetic patients found a clear correlation between the decline in glycaemic control and atorvastatin intake (8).

Statin users had a 46% higher chance of developing new-onset diabetes with a stark 24% increase in insulin resistance accompanied by a 12% decreased insulin secretion (6). Statins essentially work by lowering the synthesis of products in the mevalonate pathway, thereby leading to a significant increase in the loading of cholesterol which directly causes impairment in the performance of beta cells, causing a drop in insulin sensitivity (6). There is no doubt that hyperlipidemia is linked to the onset of cardiovascular disorders and type 2 diabetes and that statins help in lowering the lipid content (7). But little doubt also remains that statins result in new-onset diabetes. This directly translates to the fact that traditional medicine has been overstated in its ability to cure ailments because the underlying conditions are not solved holistically. The human body is a complex whole of different interconnected mechanisms. All of these metabolic processes are essential to driving the biological being.

Anomalies in human health could, therefore, be due to one or more than one often associated reason. Traditional commonplace medicines, like statins, fix one aspect of the problem, often ignoring the bigger picture and misjudged impact on the associated pathways. Contemporary medicine strongly advocates for personalized treatment, which takes into account the patient's predisposition to ailments such as diabetes, for example, family history of cardiovascular complications, obesity, metabolic syndrome, and psychological stressors. Only then is a treatment proposed by a multi-disciplinary team of professionals belonging to different scientific specialties. Other advances in the research and development forte include using patient-derived proliferating stem cells to form three-dimensional organoids for directly testing response to certain drugs (9). These approaches help to identify and answer the most fundamental alterations in the functioning of a certain or pathway.

3. What is the rate of prescriptions in the United States as it compares to other countries.

About 200 million people or more worldwide take statins for controlling cholesterol and protecting against cardiovascular complications (11). In 2003, statins were hailed as the most sold pharmaceutical drug throughout medical history. In 2005, they sold for $18.7 billion in the United States (11). In 2016, with a significant reduction in retail price due to patent expiry, sales exponentially increased by 60%. In 2018, 35 million people in the US were prescribed statins (11). In the UK, only 7 to 8 million people are actively consuming statins. The ongoing COVID-19 pandemic also saw the ever-increasing popularity of statins for the treatment of hospitalized patients due to its immuno-modulatory properties (10).

From 2020 to 2027, the statin industry is expected to grow at a compound annual growth rate of 3.70% (11). One of the reasons for this projected rate is the increasingly sedentary lifestyles of general population and lack of physical exercise, which causes cholesterol build up. Statins, however, have been repeatedly implicated in causing neuropathy, compromising muscular and cardiac strength. In diabetic patients, statins have been found to decrease cholesterol levels but with a simultaneous increase in neuropathic pain.

4. Is there a clear correlation between statin medication and the reduction of cardiovascular disease and mortality.

Statins are known to protect against cardiovascular complications and reduce mortality by 12%, but they do so at the expense of other metabolic processes (12). A study compared the efficacy of statins and a Mediterranean diet to improve mortality and protect against diabetes, cardiovascular complications, and cancer using secondary research (13). They debunked not only the overstated benefits of statins but also the myth that merely lowering cholesterol helps protect against coronary heart disease (13).

Another study, however, inferred that the controversy continues to propagate because a standard method of ascertaining the adverse effects of statins does not exist (14). The above discussion easily maintains that the medical side effects outweigh the benefits. An all-encompassing treatment plan is needed to meet the body's requirements without offsetting metabolic and physiological balance. In this regard, it is also crucial to mention the effect of increased statin intake and its pathophysiology on muscular and cardiac health and implications in neuropathy.

5. What are the side effects of statins and how do they relate to the skeletal system?

In the skeletal muscle system, statins have been reported to cause muscle soreness, cramping, myopathy, weakness, myalgia, and fatigue (15). In severe cases, increased statin use can cause rhabdomyolysis in which rapid muscle degradation can lead to death (16). All these conditions have been found by scientists to be dose-dependent (15, 16). Conditions such as renal or hepatic disease increase the patient's susceptibility to statin-induced myopathy.

The problem with these identifications is that they are not readily detectable and are not considered standard. They are rare conditions, in need of proper monitoring strategies to be classified explicitly as statin-induced anomalies. Studying disease pathophysiology indicates that statin-induced muscle degeneration is multifactorial, which means that it affects multiple metabolic processes and pathways such as central dogma, protein synthesis, and signal transduction mechanisms (17). Disturbance in these pathways coupled with a predisposition to metabolic dysfunction exacerbates myopathy (17). Although cholesterol is the primary target of statins, it also directly hamper the action of coenzyme Q10, which is directly involved in the healthy functioning of a skeletal muscle (16).

6. What are the side effects of statin on our muscular strength?

Muscular strength is also adversely affected by statin use. Muscle soreness after exercise is particularly ignored and downplayed, but studies have shown that muscle injury after exercise is particularly exacerbated due to statin use (18, 17, 19). Creatinine Kinase levels in serum are used as biomarkers to measure muscle damage (17). Patients who exercised and took statins were found to have a higher percentage of serum Creatinine Kinase suggesting increased muscle damage as compared to patients who exercised with the same intensity but did not take statins (18).

Moreover, non-statin users have a higher mean leg strength as compared to statin users. These observations were made on follow-up patients, while studies in rats indicated that many of the statin drugs did not lower mean leg strength (15). The data is, therefore, suggestive and requires more research to not only elucidate clear mechanisms of action leading to muscle weakness but also to categorize the severity of muscle-related side effects brought on by statins in a dose-dependent manner. This will help to devise future treatment plans concerning cholesterol control, keeping in close consideration the muscle-related side effects of statins.

7. What are the side effects of statins on our heart strength?

The primary function of statins is to restore cardiac function by removing cholesterol and protecting against cardiovascular diseases (21). These cardiovascular diseases include hypertension, heart failure, and other heart diseases. They lower the risk of heart failure and stroke by getting rid of fatty plaques (20, 21). There is as such no evidence of adverse effects brought on by statins on cardiac muscle strength. Statins are the first choice to protect against cardiovascular complications, particularly in individuals who are predisposed because of obesity and family history. Statins help in improving endothelial properties and function, they prevent platelets from aggregating, clot formation, and help to reduce oxidative damage and inflammation (20). The Jupiter and Asteroid Trials, which were large studies based on random sampling, established that patients taking statins were significantly protected against cardiovascular complications as compared to patients who were not taking statins (22, 23).

8. What impact do statins have on peripheral neuropathy?

Statin users are 14 times more susceptible to peripheral neuropathy (24). This happens primarily because statins obstruct the mitochondrial oxidative pathway by affecting Coenzyme Q10's function (24). Patients with type 2 diabetes are susceptible to develop peripheral neuropathy, which is exacerbated with statin use. This side effect happens in a dose-dependent manner. Some studies postulate that it is, actually, the statin-induced peripheral neuropathy that is masquerading as autoimmune polyneuropathy observed in diabetes (25).

Patients with peripheral neuropathy experience burning or tingling sensations. Peripheral neuropathy affects nerves in the limbs (26). Primary treatment options include keeping glucose levels in the desired range and taking care of the feet. Drug-induced neuropathy is seen to develop more frequently in people who are predisposed to it with a condition such as diabetes or genetic influence (24, 25, 26, 27). In any case, to confirm the efficacy of treatment, it is important to devise new and more sensitive techniques of neuromodulation (27). Early detection of disease onset and controlling of causative elements such as glucose levels help in further disease progress.

The efficacy of medication to control peripheral neuropathy is still debatable, and lifestyle changes are recommended for prevention and protection (26). In essence, the majority of the studies looking into the effect of statins in inducing peripheral neuropathy to establish a potent link between the disease and dose-dependent drug usage. Regardless of these evidence-based insights, the market projection continues to foresee an increase in the statin market (11).

The above discussion highlights that traditionally popular medications such as statins are not a solution but instead provide temporary relief to one problem while aggravating other conditions such as peripheral neuropathy and skeletal muscle damage. Their paradoxical behavior in the human body has led to a serious debate regarding their long-term effects. Medical treatments need to think of the fundamental needs of the human body without eliciting serious damage. So far, the debate and scientific evidence are against the long-term use of heavy dosage statin drugs, but the increasing trend in sedentary lifestyles has increased the cause of concern for high cholesterol levels. These high levels of cholesterol mean that statins are here to stay in the market despite their negative consequences.

9. How does homocysteine play a role in the detection of cardiovascular disease as compared to LDL cholesterol?

Cardiovascular diseases (CVD) are multi-factorial, meaning that there can be multiple causative agents, making them harder to predict and detect accurately. There have been several reports since the 1990s which cite homocysteine, an intermediate amino acid formed during the biosynthesis of methionine and cysteine, as a risk factor for CVD (28). Some researchers, however, argue that homocysteine cannot be causally correlated with CVD and that classical risk factors like dyslipidemia account for more than one-third of CVD events (29).

However, there have been recent reports that correlate high levels of homocysteine with a greater risk of CVD (30). Hyperhomocyste-inemia, which is the elevation of homocysteine in blood plasma due to environmental and genetic factors, can cause cell damage rigidity of vascular tissue and dyshomeostasis, which collectively contribute to CVD. Baszczuk et al. (2014) found that people with hyperhomocysteinemia had elevated HDL and LDL cholesterol levels concurrently with hypertension and therefore a greater risk for developing CVD (31). Sahu et al. (2015) empirically demonstrated that homocysteine sensitivity and accuracy were better than other classic biomarkers and risk factors (32).

The evidence in support of homocysteine as an essential factor in CVD has been compiling over the years since the late 20th century. While one factor cannot possibly describe a complicated set of disorders like CVD, it can certainly aid in expanding the toolkit required for proper diagnosis and prevention. Because of this reason and the mounting evidence in its support, homocysteine concentration can be established as a new biomarker in addition to classic biomarkers such as HDL and LDL cholesterol levels to improve the predictive power of cardiovascular diseases.

10. What is an effective approach to reducing homocysteine levels?

While it can be an effective biomarker for the detection of CVD, it is ultimately implicated in the progression of the disease. However, hyperhomocysteinemia can be reversed with certain therapeutic strategies. The goal of these therapeutic agents is to either convert the amino acid to cysteine or methionine (33). Dietary supplements like Vitamin B and Folic acid are generally used to remethylate homocysteine to methionine and have been shown to reduce homocysteine concentrations by 32% if taken concurrently (34). Follow-up studies have strived to ascertain if the lowering of homocysteine could indirectly decrease the risk of CVD. A 2006 clinical trial found that such is not the case, and while dietary supplements lowered homocysteine levels, they could not reduce the risk of CVD (35).

A meta-analysis of large-scale clinical trials by Clark et al. (2011) also revealed that there is no causal relationship between homocysteine levels reduction and CVD risk. Over five years in various studies, it was seen that lowering of homocysteine levels via dietary supplements did not have any benefits in CVD outcomes in 35,603 participants. In addition to this, there have been reports that correlate the risk of developing cancer with a prolonged uptake of folic acid (36).

This poses a dilemma questioning the results of these studies, which perhaps did not examine any underlying factors that could have contributed to homocysteine levels not correlating with CVD risk. This affirms a notion that vitamin B complex and folic acid cannot be taken as daily supplements in patients with a high risk of CVD as they provide no perceptible advantage over a control group. There is evidence to suggest that homocysteine is more closely associated with renal function, which was not considered in the aforementioned studies (44). So, while dietary supplements can reduce homocysteine levels, a better therapeutic target could relate CVD with renal impairment.

11. What is an effective alternative to reduce cholesterol without the use of statin medication?

There are several over-the-counter alternatives to statin. One of the more common ones is niacin, which has been empirically demonstrated to decrease the secretion of LDL by inhibiting its precursor. In addition to this, niacin can inhibit the secretion of triglycerides and HDL cholesterol as well. However, a controversial study in 2014 found that long-term administration of niacin led to an increased risk of strokes and hyperglycemia (37). Nevertheless, niacin is an FDA-approved drug with formulations ranging from immediate, extended, and sustained release. A protein inhibitor named Ezetimibe blocks cholesterol absorption from the gastrointestinal tract and has been shown to bear a 17% reduction in LDL levels in patients suffering from hyperlipidemia (38). Its effects on the risk of CVD have been studied in a recent clinical trial IMPROVE-IT; however, it is currently used as an adjunct to simvastatin (39).

Fabric acid is another alternative that has been demonstrated to decrease LDL and increase HDL cholesterol. It is not without its side effects, however, with fibrates causing dyspepsia and gallstones (40). Bile acid sequestrants which sequester bile acid into an insoluble form later ejected from the body, help lower the level of bile acids in the liver. This, in turn, causes an increased conversion of LDL to bile acids, thereby also increasing HDL and triglyceride levels. While it can be used as an alternative, the efficacy is a low 30% as compared to statins (41). A more promising candidate for a potential replacement for statins is the antibody to a serine protease PCSK9 which can then be used to decrease the concentration of LDL. Two such antibodies, alirocumab, and evolocumab have been shown to reduce LDL concentration significantly and have good safety profiles as well (42, 43).

Their comparative efficacy with statins has not yet been established, but they remain good candidates for statin-free therapies. It is evident that while there are existing alternatives to statins, they do not have the same therapeutic efficacy. In some cases, these alternatives may also cause side effects similar to or worse than statins. Except for perhaps PCSK9, the usage of the rest of the alternatives in clinical settings as a reliable replacement for statins remains debatable.

References

1. Gallaghar, P. (2019). *Statins review 'urgently needed to find out if millions benefit*. News. Available at:

https://inews.co.uk/news/health/statins-review-nhs-government-chief-medical-adviser-norman-lamb-333188 (Accessed: 14 July 2021).

2. Malhotra, A. (2019) Do statins really work? Who benefits? Who has the power to cover up the side effects?, *European Scientist*. Available at: https://www.europeanscientist.com/en/features/do-statins-really-work-who-benefits-who-has-the-power-to-cover-up-the-side-effects/#_ftn1 (Accessed: 14 July 2021).

3. Barter, P. J., Cochran, B. J., & Rye, K.-A. (2018). *CETP inhibition, statins and diabetes. Atherosclerosis*. 278, 143-146.

4. Paseban, M., Butler, A. E., & Sahebkar, A. (2019). Mechanisms of statin-induced new-onset diabetes. *Journal of Cellular Physiology*. 1-11.

5. Brault, M., Ray, J., Gomez, Y.-H., Mantzoros, C. S., & Daskalopoulou, S. S. (2014). Statin treatment and new-onset diabetes: A review of proposed mechanisms. *Metabolism: Clinical and Experimental*, 63(6), 735–745.

6. Carmena, R., & Betteridge, D. J. (2019). Diabetogenic Action of Statins: Mechanisms. *Current Atherosclerosis Reports, 21(6)*.

7. Yu, Q., Chen, Y., & Xu, C.-B. (2017). Statins and New-Onset Diabetes Mellitus: LDL Receptor May Provide a Key Link. *Frontiers in Pharmacology*, 8(372).

8. Angelidi, A. M., Stambolliu, E., Adamapoulou, K. I., & Kousoulis, A. A. (2018). Is atorvastatin associated with new-onset diabetes or deterioration of glycemic control? Systematic

review using data from 1.9 million patients. *Int J Endocrinol.* 2018;2018:8380192.

9. Lin, A., Sved Skottvoll, F., Rayner, S., Pedersen-Bjergaard, S., Sullivan, G., Krauss, S., Ray Wilson, S. and Harrison, S., (2020). 3D cell culture models and organ-on-a-chip: Meet separation science and mass spectrometry. *Electrophoresis, 41*(1-2), pp.56-64.

10. Pal R, Banerjee M, Yadav U, Bhattacharjee, S. (2021). Statin use and clinical outcomes in patients with COVID-19: An updated systematic review and meta-analysis. *BMJ. Postgraduate Medical Journal. 0; 1-6.*

11. Data Bridge (2021). *Statin Market – Global Industry Trends and Forecast to 2027 | Data Bridge Market Research* (2021). Available at: https://www.databridgemarketresearch.com/reports/global-statin-market (Accessed: 20 July 2021).

12. Ray, K. K., Seshasai, S. R. K., and Erqou, S., (2019) Statins and All-Cause Mortality in High-Risk Primary Prevention: A Meta-analysis of 11 Randomized Controlled Trials Involving 65 229 Participants. *Arch Intern Med.*170(12):1024–1031.

13. DuBroff, R., & de Lorgeril, M. (2015). Cholesterol confusion and statin controversy. *World Journal of Cardiology, 7*(7), 404–409. https://doi.org/10.4330/wjc.v7.i7.404

14. Mansi, I., Mortensen, E., (2013). The controversy of a wider statin utilization: why? Expert Opinion. *Drug Saf*;12(3):327-37. DOI: 10.1517/14740338.2013.779667.

15. Ananthakumar, A., Liu, Y., Fernandez, C. E., Truskey, G. A., & Voora, D. (2020). Modeling statin myopathy in a human

skeletal muscle microphysiological system. *PloS one, 15*(11), e0242422.

16. Allard, N. A., Schirris, T. J., Verheggen, R. J., Russel, F. G., Rodenburg, R. J., Smeitink, J. A., ... & Timmers, S. (2018). Statins affect skeletal muscle performance: evidence for disturbances in energy metabolism. *The Journal of Clinical Endocrinology & Metabolism, 103*(1), 75-84.

17. Bouitbir, J., Sanvee, G. M., Panajatovic, M. V., Singh, F., & Krähenbühl, S. (2020). Mechanisms of statin-associated skeletal muscle-associated symptoms. *Pharmacological Research, 154*, 104201.

18. Morville, T., Dohlmann, T. L., Kuhlman, A. B., Sahl, R. E., Kriegbaum, M., Larsen, S., ... & Helge, J. W. (2019). Aerobic exercise performance and muscle strength in statin users—the LIFESTAT study. *Medicine & Science in Sports & Exercise, 51*(7), 1429-1437.

19. Taylor, B. A., & Thompson, P. D. (2018). Statin-associated muscle disease: advances in diagnosis and management. *Neurotherapeutics, 15*(4), 1006-1017.

20. Tian, X. Q., Yang, Y. J., Li, Q., Xu, J., Huang, P. S., Xiong, Y. Y., ... & Geng, Y. J. (2019). Combined therapy with atorvastatin and atorvastatin-pretreated mesenchymal stem cells enhances cardiac performance after acute myocardial infarction by activating the SDF-1/CXCR4 axis. *American journal of translational research, 11*(7), 4214.

21. Tian, X. Q., Yang, Y. J., Li, Q., Xu, J., Huang, P. S., Xiong, Y. Y., ... & Geng, Y. J. (2019). Combined therapy with

atorvastatin and atorvastatin-pretreated mesenchymal stem cells enhances cardiac performance after acute myocardial infarction by activating the SDF-1/CXCR4 axis. *American journal of translational research, 11*(7), 4214.

22. Khera, A. V., Demler, O. V., Adelman, S. J., Collins, H. L., Glynn, R. J., Ridker, P. M., ... & Mora, S. (2017). Cholesterol efflux capacity, high-density lipoprotein particle number, and incident cardiovascular events: an analysis from the JUPITER Trial (Justification for the Use of Statins in Prevention: An Intervention Trial Evaluating Rosuvastatin). *Circulation, 135*(25), 2494-2504.

23. Susekov, A. V. (2021). Statin therapy and atherosclerosis regression. *Cardiovascular Therapy and Prevention, 9*(7), 112-117.

24. Özdemir, I. H., Copkiran, Ö., Tıkız, H., & Tıkız, C. (2019). Peripheral polyneuropathy in patients receiving long-term statin therapy. *Turk Kardiyol Dern Ars, 47*(7), 554-563.

25. Emad, M., Arjmand, H., Farpour, H. R., & Kardeh, B. (2018). Lipid-lowering drugs (statins) and peripheral neuropathy. *Electronic physician, 10*(3), 6527.

26. Mulchandani, R., Lyngdoh, T., & Kakkar, A. K. (2020). Statin use and safety concerns: an overview of the past, present, and the future. *Expert Opinion on Drug Safety, 19*(8), 1011-1024.

27. Bloomingdale, P., & Mager, D. E. (2019). Machine learning models for the prediction of chemotherapy-induced peripheral neuropathy. *Pharmaceutical Research, 36*(2), 35.

28. Shenoy, V., Mehendale, V., Prabhu, K., Shetty, R. and Rao, P., 2014. Correlation of serum homocysteine levels with the severity of coronary artery disease. *Indian Journal of Clinical Biochemistry, 29*(3), pp.339-344.

29. Faeh, D., Chiolero, A. and Paccaud, F., 2006. Homocysteine as a risk factor for cardiovascular disease: should we (still) worry about it?. *Swiss medical weekly, 136*(47-48), pp.745-756.

30. Okura, T., Miyoshi, K.I., Irita, J., Enomoto, D., Nagao, T., Kukida, M., Tanino, A., Kudo, K., Pei, Z. and Higaki, J., 2014. Hyperhomocysteinemia is one of the risk factors associated with cerebrovascular stiffness in hypertensive patients, especially elderly males. *Scientific reports, 4*(1), pp.1-5.

31. Baszczuk, A., Musialik, K., Kopczyński, J., Thielemann, A., Kopczyński, Z., Kęsy, L. and Dopierała, G., 2014. Hyperhomocysteinemia, lipid and lipoprotein disturbances in patients with primary hypertension. *Advances in Medical Sciences, 59*(1), pp.68-73.

32. Sahu, A., Gupta, T., Kavishwar, A. and Singh, R.K., 2015. Cardiovascular diseases risk prediction by homocysteine in comparison to other markers: a study from Madhya Pradesh. *J Assoc Physicians India, 63*(10), pp.37-40.

33. Mujawar, S.A., Patil, V.W. and Daver, R.G., 2011. Study of serum homocysteine, folic acid and vitamin B 12 in patients with preeclampsia. *Indian journal of clinical biochemistry, 26*(3), pp.257-260.

34. Clarke, R., Halsey, J., Bennett, D. and Lewington, S., 2011. Homocysteine and vascular disease: review of published results of the homocysteine-lowering trials. *Journal of inherited metabolic disease, 34*(1), pp.83-91.

35. Blankenberg, S., McQueen, M.J., Smieja, M., Pogue, J., Balion, C., Lonn, E., Rupprecht, H.J., Bickel, C., Tiret, L., Cambien, F. and Gerstein, H., 2006. Comparative impact of multiple biomarkers and N-Terminal pro-brain natriuretic peptide in the context of conventional risk factors for the prediction of recurrent cardiovascular events in the Heart Outcomes Prevention Evaluation (HOPE) Study. Circulation, 114(3), pp.201-208.

36. Figueiredo, J.C., Grau, M.V., Haile, R.W., Sandler, R.S., Summers, R.W., Bresalier, R.S., Burke, C.A., McKeown-Eyssen, G.E. and Baron, J.A., 2009. Folic acid and risk of prostate cancer: results from a randomized clinical trial. *Journal of the National Cancer Institute, 101*(6), pp.432-435.

37. Toth, P.P., Murthy, A.M., Sidhu, M.S. and Boden, W.E., 2015. Is HPS2-THRIVE the death knell for niacin?. *Journal of clinical lipidology, 9*(3), pp.343-350.

38. Dujovne, C.A., Ettinger, M.P., McNeer, J.F., Lipka, L.J., LeBeau, A.P., Suresh, R., Yang, B., Veltri, E.P. and Ezetimibe Study Group, 2002. Efficacy and safety of a potent new selective cholesterol absorption inhibitor, Ezetimibe, in patients with primary hypercholesterolemia. *The American journal of cardiology, 90*(10), pp.1092-1097.

39. Murphy, S.A., Cannon, C.P., Blazing, MA, Giugliano, R.P., White, J.A., Lokhnygina, Y., Reist, C., I'm, K., Bohula, E.A.,

Isaza, D. and Lopez-Sendon, J., 2016. Reduction in total cardiovascular events with ezetimibe/simvastatin post-acute coronary syndrome: the IMPROVE-IT trial. *Journal of the American College of Cardiology*, *67*(4), pp.353-361.

40. Shattat, G.F., 2015. A review article on hyperlipidemia: types, treatments and new drug targets. *Biomedical and Pharmacology Journal*, *7*(1), pp.399-409.

41. Staels, B. and Fonseca, V.A., 2009. Bile acids and metabolic regulation: mechanisms and clinical responses to bile acid sequestration. *Diabetes care*, *32*(suppl 2), pp.S237-S245.

42. Stein, E.A., Gipe, D., Bergeron, J., Gaudet, D., Weiss, R., Dufour, R., Wu, R. and Pordy, R., 2012. Effect of a monoclonal antibody to PCSK9, REGN727/SAR236553, to reduce low-density lipoprotein cholesterol in patients with heterozygous familial hypercholesterolaemia on stable statin dose with or without ezetimibe therapy: a phase 2 randomised controlled trial. *The Lancet*, *380*(9836), pp.29-36.

43. Sheridan, C., 2013. Phase 3 data for PCSK9 inhibitor wows. *Nature Biotechnology*, *31*(12), pp.1057-1059.

44. Spence, J.D., 2013. B vitamin therapy for homocysteine: renal function and vitamin B12 determine cardiovascular outcomes. *Clinical chemistry and laboratory medicine*, *51*(3), pp.633-637.

Chapter 12

OVERALL BENEFITS OF A CLASS
IV LASER FOR NEUROPATHY

L ight has for thousands of years been recognized as an energy
with therapeutic effects. Today, this information has evolved
into the use of laser devices and machines that can send controlled amounts of lights into your cells as a form of treatment. The
light treatment process does not address only disease symptoms but
also treats the root causes of those diseases. In general, light therapy
has been found to provide long-term therapeutic benefits to patients.

Laser therapy can be described as a medical treatment that light to
bring about health effects in a tissue. It employs a specific wavelength
of focused light in medical science to interact with tissues and stimulate the process of photobiomodulation (PBM) or photobiostimulation.
Photobiomodulation is the process by which electromagnetic energy
in form of protons, is introduced into a cell or tissue. Within the cell
or tissue, these protons interact chemically and biologically with the
cytochrome c complex in the cells' mitochondria. This interaction pro-
ceeds to yield therapeutic effects.

This use of electromagnetic energy is not new to our bodies. The cells and tissues in our bodies naturally use this energy to fuel their actions and carry out physiological functions. These include the production of beats by the heart, sending of signals by the brain, nerve stimulation, and cellular metabolism.

Compared to other lines of treatment such as drugs and surgery, light or laser therapy has been proven to aid natural body healing through photochemical processes. Other benefits of laser therapy include reduction and relief of pain, reduction in inflammation, decrease in muscle spasm, promotion of wound healing, tissue regeneration, immuno-modulation, increase in cellular metabolism, increased range of motion, and improvement in body blood microcirculation, amongst others.

The use of laser devices has been proven to be safe, has little to no side effects, is specific, convenient, and quick in providing treatment without drugs or surgery. It has also been cleared by the FDA as a non-invasive, non-pharmacological treatment for pain relief. Research shows that it is equally effective as other forms of rehabilitation and in some cases, more.

What is Class IV Laser?

Lasers are classified into eight classes according to how much harm the laser beam can cause. These are classes I, I Product. IM, II, IIM, IIIR, IIIB, and IV. Class IV laser ranks the highest in classes of lasers and is the most hazardous class of laser radiation. It is high-powered in terms of wavelength, power, energy, and pulse duration. It is mostly used in medical practice for surgical and cosmetic purposes.

However, it is hazardous to the eye. In order words, prolonged exposure can cause harm to your eye and result in eye damage. Class IV lasers are powerful enough to burn and cause significant harm to your skin. Hence, your eyes and skin must be protected from direct or reflected light from direct laser beams or scattered beams. Class IV lasers can potentially burn materials within close range, particularly lightweight and/or dark materials. If not appropriately handled, class IV lasers can result in a fire incident and produce poisonous fumes.

Class IV lasers could be visible or non-visible. There are only four classes of visible-beam lasers- class II, class IIIR, class IIIB, and class IV. The power output or continuous wave (CW) of visible-light class IV lasers is 0.5 watts or 500mW and above. In pulse systems, these lasers can produce more than 125mJ below 0.25 seconds.

Hence, class IV laser therapy is the use of high-powered laser light focused and sent into tissues to reduce pain, swelling, and inflammation, and boost healing.

Differences between Class IV Laser Therapy and Cold Laser Therapy

Cold laser therapy is a light therapy that uses Class IIIB lasers. In medical practice, they are limited in use as opposed to class IV lasers. The following are differences between class IV lasers and cold (class IIIB) lasers and/or laser therapy.

	Class IV therapy	Cold laser therapy
Description	Use of high-powered, intense devices.	Use of "low-powered, LLLT (low-level laser therapy), cold laser' devices.
Power output	The minimum power output of laser used is 500mW or 0.5W	The minimum power output is 5mW and the maximum power output of the laser used is 500mW or 0.5W
Wavelength	The most recommended primary wavelength for treatment is either 810nm or 980nm.	The wavelength used for the treatment ranges from 600nm to 980m.
Range in medical practice	Wide range, used in medical, surgical, cosmetic, and military purposes.	Limited range, used for wounds, superficial lesions, to relieve pain and swelling, reduce fat, improve circulation, etc. If used for other deep tissue and musculoskeletal problems, a long period of treatment is required which is not recommended in medical practice.
Time to yield therapeutic effects	Yields therapeutic effects within the shortest time possible.	Takes more time to yield therapeutic effects compared to class IV therapy.
Treatment surface area	Covers up to 77cm² treatment surface area	Covers treatment surface area of 0.3cm² to 5.0cm²
Hazard potential	Class IV laser poses a severe hazard risk to the eye, skin, and materials. Also, poses a fire risk.	Cold laser poses hazard risk (lower than Class IV laser) to the eye and skin.
Effect of laser used on the eye	Can damage your eye instantly if you stare at the laser dot.	Can damage the eye if you stare at the laser dot for many seconds within close range.
Production of diffuse reflections	Class IV lasers can produce diffuse reflections that are as hazardous as the light beams themselves	Cold lasers do not produce diffuse reflections, except for high-power class IIIB lasers.

Nominal ocular hazard distance (the distance between the unobstructed laser beam and the eye. Do not stay within this distance)	733ft (224m) for light beams that have a power output of 1000mW or 1W. 2320ft (710m) for light beams that have a power output of 10000mW or 10W	520ft (160m) for light beams that have a power output of 499.9mW
Effect of laser used on the skin	Class IV laser can burn the skin instantly.	Cold laser can heat the skin if the light beam is held at close range to the skin and long enough.
Effect of laser used on materials	Class IV laser can burn materials instantly.	Cold laser can burn materials if light beams are held long and close enough to them.
Control required	Requires significant control	Require specific control

Advantages of Class IV Therapy over Cold Laser Therapy

The use of cold laser therapy in medical practice is limited because of low energy, low dosage, and poor penetration. This is in comparison with the class IV therapy. Hence, advantages of class IV therapy over cold laser therapy include the following:

Higher amounts of therapeutic energy and faster treatment time

Class IV laser therapy provides higher wattage of therapeutic energy to cells and tissues, thus ensuring better positive outcomes. The higher the amount of energy delivered, the shorter and faster the treatment time. Compared to cold laser therapy, class IV laser therapy delivers up to 1,500 more energy to treat pain and other medical conditions.

Greater power density

Class IV laser therapy does not only produce more power output but more concentration of the power output. With more power density, more therapeutic outcomes are achieved.

Continuous power supply

With class IV lasers, you enjoy a continuous power supply and light can pass through the probe throughout the total operating time. This is unlike cold lasers where the power is pulsed half of the time, hence light can only be passed for half of the operating time.

Consistent dose of energy

Usually, class IV lasers deliver a steady and constant amount of energy over a given treatment period.

Deeper penetration into tissues

Class IV laser therapy provides a deeper depth of penetration into body cells, tissues, and organs within the shortest time possible. While class III lasers can penetrate depths of $0.5cm^2$ to $2.0cm^2$, class IV laser therapy provides deep tissue penetration up to $10cm^2$. This penetration provides effective tissue healing.

Wider treatment surface area

Class IV laser therapy covers more treatment surface area than cold laser therapy. This makes it the best option for areas like hips, lumbar spine, and quadriceps. Cold lasers cover treatment areas from $0.3cm^2$ to $5.0cm^2$ while class IV laser therapy covers up to $77cm^2$ of treatment surface area.

Superior fiber optic cables

Fiber optic cables transmit light energy from the laser to the probe. Class IV lasers have fiber optic cables of better quality and function than cold lasers where up to 50 percent of the energy produced could get lost before it gets to the end of the probe.

The Science behind Class IV Laser Therapy

Class IV laser therapy works via the process called photobiomodulation (PBM). During PBM, electromagnetic energy, that is protons are introduced into the cell or tissue in the body and interact with the cells' mitochondria. This interaction generates biological and chemical reactions that bring about therapeutic effects such as pain relief, inflammation reduction, muscle relaxation, and tissue repair, amongst others. Factors that determine photobiomodulation include:

- Type of light
- Light wavelength
- Operating modes
- Power

In class IV laser therapy, the wavelength length of the laser provides deeper penetration depth than other classes of laser radiation. Hence, energy enters into deep tissues, nerves, ligaments, tendons, and muscle tissue in lesser time. Therapy sessions last between 2-6 minutes and provide for more and larger treatment surface areas to be treated.

Class IV laser therapy stimulates several photochemical processes including:

- Stimulation of cytochrome c
- Generation of ATP
- Accelerated DNA and RNA synthesis
- Increased collagen synthesis
- Enhanced levels of beta-endorphins and serotonin

ATP (adenosine triphosphate) production also facilitates several cellular processes including healing and regeneration processes within cells. Studies show that after class IV therapy, patients reported reduced pain, swelling, and inflammation, increased range of motion, and wound healing.

Application of Class IV Laser Therapy

Class IV laser therapy is used for the following reasons:

To reduce pain, aches, and inflammation

Class IV devices are used for patients who suffer from acute and chronic pain, and inflammation. The mode of action of these devices is photochemical, that is using light energy to stimulate chemical reactions that relieve pain, aid wound healing, and boost blood circulation. These include:

- Promoting muscle relaxation, hence, reducing pain from muscle cramps and spasms
- Reducing joint pain and stiffness
- Reducing arthritic pain symptoms
- Improving blood circulation
- Treating post-surgical wounds and pain

To recover from injuries (acute and chronic)

Class IV laser therapy is used to treat acute and chronic injuries. Examples include tendonitis, strains, and sprains. These injuries also result in pain and inflammation and hence, laser therapy comes in handy in treating both pain, swelling, and other signs of inflammation, as well as aid treating.

Recovery can also be boosted by stimulating immune system response, nerve regeneration, and muscle relaxation.

To treat skin disorders including scars, burns, wounds, etc.

Class IV laser therapy can promote the healing of several skin conditions such as wounds, lesions, burns, and scars. Surgical incisions can also benefit from laser therapy, as it also reduces the risk for infections.

To treat neuropathy

Neuropathy is a term used to describe nerve damage. Nerve damage can bring about symptoms such as pain, muscle cramps and spasm, tingling sensation, numbness, loss of function, and bone degeneration. These symptoms can be relieved by administering class IV laser therapy.

To treat cancer

Class IV laser therapy can also be used to shrink or kill tumors, polyps, or precancerous growths. For patients with cancer, they can be used to relieve cancer symptoms. It can also be used to prevent the spread of tumor cells by sealing lymph vessels.

To improve vision

Laser therapy can be used to improve vision. Studies have shown that laser therapy may be sued to repair a detached retina, hence improving vision.

For cosmetic purposes

In the cosmetic industry and medical practice, class IV lasers can be used to erase birthmarks, sun spots, stretch marks, wrinkles, scars, and blemishes. They can be used to remove hair and tattoos.

Others include:

- To treat hair loss associated with alopecia or aging

- To remove parts of the prostate
- To treat kidney stones
- To close up blood vessels and stop or prevent bleeding
- To close up lymph vessels to prevent swelling

Benefits of Class IV Laser Therapy

The following are benefits offered by class IV therapy. They include:

- Treatment causes less or no pain
- Easily applied
- Drug-free
- Surgery free
- No side or adverse effects
- Non-invasive
- Highly effective for several diseases and conditions
- Affordable
- Non-toxic
- No drug interactions
- Treatment is an alternative option for patients who have undergone other therapies that failed
- Has long-lasting results

Conditions that Class IV Laser Therapy can treat

Class IV laser therapy has been shown to treat numerous health conditions. They include:

- Peripheral neuropathy
- Diabetic neuropathy
- Headaches and migraines

- Neck injury and pain
- Back pain
- TMJ
- Arthritis pain (could be knee, hip, shoulder, etc.)
- Sciatic pain
- Bruises
- Fibromyalgia
- Carpal Tunnel syndrome
- Bursitis
- Bulging, Herniated, or Disc Protrusion
- Plantar Fasciitis
- Epicondylitis (tennis elbow)
- Tendinitis
- Runners knee (patellofemoral pain syndrome)
- Bunion pain
- Diabetic ulcers
- Trigger fingers
- Burns
- Contusions
- Skin conditions like wounds and scars
- Sports injuries
- Auto injuries
- Work-related injuries
- Acute pain related to post-surgical recovery

Class IV laser therapy can successfully conditions that are pain or inflammation-related. Others include medical conditions like kidney stones, bleeding, hair loss, and cancer.

How can a Class IV Laser Treat Neuropathy?

Neuropathy is a condition where there is nerve damage. Several conditions can cause neuropathy, however, the most common cause is diabetes. Untreated and/or poorly managed diabetes results in comprised blood circulation, reducing the supply of oxygen and nutrients to distal body parts. Once nerve damage occurs, it affects how signals are sent and received.

Unlike other tissue, nerves do not repair or regenerate. Nerve damage is irreversible, hence treatment is aimed at slowing down the progression of the neuropathy and relieving symptoms. Symptoms of neuropathy include pain, muscle cramping, bone degeneration, hypersensitivity to light, sound, and touch, and numbness or tingling sensation.

Administering laser therapy for neuropathy can help relieve pain and discomfort associated with the condition. It does this by improving blood circulation to and around the affected body parts. Usually, neuropathy occurs as a result of poor blood circulation to these areas in the first place. Hence, class IV laser therapy helps reverse that, facilitate repair, and improve nerve function by ensuring an increased supply of oxygen and nutrients to nerves in these areas. In the end, laser therapy helps to relieve neuropathic pain and discomfort.

Alongside pain relief, class IV laser neuropathy relieves other symptoms of neuropathy including reduction of inflammation, decrease in muscle cramping, and promotion of wound healing and tissue repair.

Contraindications for Class IV Laser Therapy

The contraindications for the use of therapeutic class IV laser include the following:

Over pacemakers and internal pain pumps

The use of class IV laser for therapeutic purposes over internal pacemakers is contraindicated. This is especially if the laser device uses electrical stimulation as well.

During pregnancy

Like most drugs and therapies, Class IV laser therapy should not be used on pregnant women. This is because high doses of light energy can affect the growing fetus, especially in the first trimester. While recent studies may want to include pregnant women in the therapeutic use of lasers, it is absolutely contraindicated if use will involve regions of the abdomen, low back, and pelvis.

Over the thyroid gland

The thyroid gland is a very delicate structure, and hence treatment targeted towards and around it should be done with proper caution. Studies have shown that high wattages of light radiation could bring about thyroid disorders.

Over glandular tissues

These include the thymus, ovaries, and testicles. It is believed that treatment with lasers may affect the functions of these glands and cause disorders.

In epileptics

Research shows that light (that is, pulsing visible red light with frequencies ranging from 5-10 Hz) can trigger epileptic seizures. Hence, the use of class IV lasers that produce light is contraindicated in people suffering from epilepsy. However, some can still tolerate lower frequencies.

Over growth plates in children

Class IV laser therapy is contraindicated in children, especially over bone growth plates. This however may be changing as recent studies show successful laser treatments in children.

In people living with cancer

Laser therapy could interfere with cancer treatment in patients with cancer, especially those undergoing radiation therapy

After the use of photosensitizing medications

Allowing a patient have class IV laser therapy after he or she has been given or has used photosensitizing medications is a contraindication. Examples of photosensitizing medications include antibiotics such as tetracyclines, sulfonamides, and fluoroquinolones, NSAIDs (non-steroidal anti-inflammatory drugs), and antifungals.

Diabetes

To an extent, class IV laser therapy is contraindicated in patients with diabetes. However, certain studies have shown that class IV laser therapy improved wound healing, and did not affect insulin balance in subjects with diabetes.

Direct or reflected exposure

This is a definite and absolute contraindication. Where is no adequate safety precaution taken, class IV laser therapy should be done or given. Light from class IV lasers can cause instant harm to the eyes, skin, and materials they can get in contact with. If treatment has to be given directly to or near the eye, other alternative forms of treatment should be considered. Do not also administer laser therapy over an injection site.

Others include:

- Over active epiphyses and fontanels
- Over sites of active bleeding
- When patients are wearing metallic objects or accessories such as rings, chains, and wristwatches. These should be removed and kept away or covered before the procedure.

Some of these contraindications have been termed historical. However, with recent studies showing promise, it has been recommended that laser therapy in these conditions and cases should be done with caution.

Recommended Treatment Frequency for Class IV Laser Therapy

Class IV laser therapy sessions last for about 5 to 10 minutes. This, however, depends on which areas are being treated and how large they are. Some conditions may require daily treatment, especially if conditions are characterized by significant pain levels.

Class IV laser therapy yields results within short periods. Usually, acute conditions may require 5-6 sessions for best results. On the other hand, chronic conditions may require more sessions from about 6-12 treatments. However, these are also dependent on other individual factors. There are certain conditions- terminal or life-long illnesses that may require follow-up treatment sessions, for example, 1-2 sessions every month.

The healing process also varies from person to person. Usually, you may notice your skin is dry and peeling off 5 to 7 days after laser treatment. For it to heal, it could take about 10 to 21 days depending on the condition that was treated. Usually, the healed skin is left with redness that fades within two to three months. You could also use oil-free makeup to reduce the redness.

Summary and Conclusion

Laser therapy can be described as a medical treatment that light to bring about health effects in a tissue. It employs a specific wavelength of focused light in medical science to interact with tissues and stimulate the process of photobiomodulation (PBM) or photobiostimulation. This process yields beneficial cellular reactions that result in the following: pain relief and reduction, reduction of inflammation. decrease in muscle cramping and spasm, increase in wound healing and tissue regeneration, immunomodulation, increased cellular metabolism, increased range of motion, and improvement in blood microcirculation.

Hence, class IV laser therapy is the use of high-powered laser light focused and sent into tissues to reduce pain, swelling, and inflammation, and boost healing. Class IV laser due to its high-power output and deeper depth penetration ability has shown to yield better results than cold lasers.

Contraindications however include use over glandular tissue such as the thyroid gland, testicles, ovaries, and thymus gland, over open fontanels and active epiphyses, over pacemakers and internal pain pumps, over growth plates in children, in pregnant woman, in epileptics, people with cancer and diabetes over locally injected sites, and without safety precautions in place.

Both acute and chronic conditions respond well to class IV laser therapy. Pain, swelling, and inflammation are greatly reduced. Affected areas begin optimal functioning within shorter periods compared to medical and surgical therapy. Class IV laser therapy reduces the risk for adhesions and scar tissues which can slow down the healing and recovery process. Tissue regeneration also helps restore function and strength and prevents the reoccurrence of the injury or condition.

Thus, class IV laser therapy is an effective, affordable, and alternative treatment option for acute and chronic pain and its associated symptoms.

Chapter 13

EVERYTHING YOU NEED TO KNOW ABOUT THE AUTOIMMUNE PALEO DIET

The autoimmune paleo diet, also known as the **Autoimmune Protocol** or **AIP Diet**, is a paleo diet modification that aims to heal the immune system and digestive tract lining in people with autoimmune disease. It helps to identify and eliminate nutritional triggers that may be provoking inflammation and further boosting autoimmune reactions.

Scientists refer to your gut microbiota as a group of microbial species that exist in your body. Most of these bacteria, fungi, and viruses coexist with us and do not harm us. At any given time, you have anywhere from 10 to 100 microbial cells.

Our microbiota is affected by the foods we eat, the medications we take, and our emotions. When the balance is disrupted, a disorder or a health condition might develop or worsen. Autoimmune disorders are classified as inflammatory because they overwhelm your body with white blood cells in an attempt to cure the imbalance.

The AIP diet focuses on identifying and eliminating items that promote inflammation in the gastrointestinal tract. Your digestive system cannot work normally if it is inflamed. It may result in:

- Poor nutritional absorption
- Diarrhea or vomiting
- Tenderness and discomfort in the stomach
- Cramping

If you have a metabolic or digestive health issue, you may need to avoid foods that cause sensitivities or symptoms to flare up. Some autoimmune illnesses require the elimination of foods or chemicals.

Difference From Traditional Paleo Diet:

Many people regard the AIP diet to be an extension of the paleo diet, however, it may be viewed as a stricter version of it. The AIP diet focuses on eliminating foods that people are often sensitive to reduce general inflammation. The AIP diet targets underlying inflammation in the gut, which can be a key contributor to autoimmune illness.

All grains and processed foods are excluded in the traditional Paleo diet. It emphasizes on full, nutrient-dense foods such as fruits and vegetables, organic meats, eggs, and wild-caught seafood. However, for chronic autoimmune disorders, this is frequently insufficient since not all immunological triggers are addressed.

Because the AIP diet is designed particularly for autoimmune illnesses, it is usually always essential to use it with other treatments. Herbal and nutritional supplements may be provided in addition to an autoimmune diet as part of a plan to treat you as a whole person rather than simply the disease process itself.

Benefits:

If you have been diagnosed with an autoimmune condition and wish to better control your symptoms, the autoimmune Paleo diet may be perfect for you. Its benefits include:

1-Leaky Gut:

Many people with autoimmune disorders have long-term damage to their gut barrier or lining, which leads to increased intestinal permeability, often known as leaky gut. Tight junctions in the stomach normally keep toxins and dangerous bacteria out of circulation while enabling nutrients to flow through and be carried to where they need to go in the body.

A leaky gut has damaged those tight connections, enabling poisons to 'leak' into the circulation. As a result, there is persistent inflammation and nutritional malabsorption, which may lead to the development of autoimmune disorders.

The Paleo diet for autoimmune disorders focuses on removing foods that contribute to leaky gut and replacing them with others that may help cure the gut while also reducing inflammation.

2-Inflammatory Bowel Disease:

IBD occurs when the immune system targets the linings of the intestines, resulting in diarrhea, gastrointestinal bleeding, intense bowel movements, stomach discomfort, fever, and weight loss.

According to research, adopting the autoimmune Paleo diet for three weeks may result in substantial improvements in IBD symptoms and quality of life.

3-Celiac Disease:

Celiac disease develops when the body's immune system reacts to gluten, a protein present in wheat, barley, and rye. Over time, the response causes inflammation, which destroys the intestinal lining and inhibits some nutrients from being absorbed.

A gluten-free diet is part of the treatment. Gluten, as well as other items that may lead to inflammation, are prohibited on the autoimmune Paleo diet.

4-Rheumatoid Arthritis:

In individuals with rheumatoid arthritis, the immune system creates antibodies that target the inner lining of the joints, producing swelling and inflammation. By lowering inflammation, the autoimmune Paleo diet may improve symptom management.

5-Skin Conditions Like Psoriasis And Eczema:

Autoimmune conditions, such as psoriasis and eczema, primarily affect the skin and are caused by an overactive immune system. The autoimmune Paleo diet may help persons with psoriasis or eczema improve their symptoms by identifying foods that cause inflammation.

Getting Started:

The AIP diet is divided into two parts.

1. The Elimination Phase:

The first step is an elimination phase in which foods and drugs suspected of causing gut inflammation, imbalances between good and harmful bacteria in the gut, or an immunological response are removed.

Dairy, gluten, grains, pseudo-grains (such as quinoa, buckwheat, and amaranth), legumes, nuts, seeds, nightshade vegetables, eggs, refined vegetable oils, alcohol, artificial sweeteners, food additives, and NSAIDs must be avoided for at least 30 days.

With these suspected gut irritants removed, the diet focuses on more anti-inflammatory, nutrient-dense foods like vegetables of all colors (except nightshades), well-sourced organic meat and organ meats, wild-caught fish, fermented foods, bone broths, healthy fats from avocados, olives, and coconuts, and small amounts of antioxidant-rich fruits like berries.

It also promotes the need of improving lifestyle factors including stress, sleep, and physical activity.

2. The Reintroduction Phase:

The reintroduction phase might begin after there is a noticeable improvement in symptoms and overall health. During this stage, the avoided items are progressively reintroduced into the diet, one by one, according to the person's tolerance.

The purpose of this phase is to discover which foods contribute to a person's symptoms and reintroduce those meals that do not produce symptoms while avoiding those that do. This provides us with the greatest possible nutritional variety.

Foods should be reintroduced one by one during this period, with 5–7 days in between before adding a different item. This gives a person sufficient time to observe whether any of their symptoms return before proceeding with the reintroduction procedure.

Following the diet's elimination phase, you reintroduce excluded food categories one by one and analyze your response. If a response develops, these foods should be reintroduced. The tolerance should be tested again at a later time (usually at least after another month of removal from the diet). The autoimmune protocol (AIP) diet assists in the discovery of a more tailored paleo-based diet that reduces inflammation, promotes gut healing, and reduces autoimmune-related symptoms over time.

Foods To Eat:

In an autoimmune Paleo diet following person should consume:

- Any vegetables, excluding those from the nightshade family; and high-quality fish rich in omega-3 fatty acids.
- Fermented foods
- Low portions of fruit oils such as olive, coconut, and avocado oils
- Lean meats and liver.
- In general, the diet includes whole foods that are free of additives such as sugar.

Foods To Avoid:

When following an AIP diet, you should avoid the following food groups:

- Tomatoes, potatoes, peppers, and eggplants

- Grains
- Legumes
- Dairy products with vegetable oils
- Coffee
- Coffee
- Seeds and nuts
- Alcohol,
- Food additives such as refined or added sugars

Short Term And Long Term Effects Of Autoimmune Paleo Diet:

While the autoimmune paleo diet can help with losing weight, blood pressure control, and blood sugar control in the short term, experts warn that in the long run, this eating style may lead to vitamin shortages and other potential health issues.

If you're thinking about trying the autoimmune paleo diet, the first problem you'll probably face is dealing with low energy levels. You may feel fatigued and irritable if you do not consume enough energy-rich carbohydrates. If you're used to eating carb-heavy foods like bread and spaghetti, those unpleasant emotions may be considerably worse.

Switching to an autoimmune paleo diet, according to studies, results in short-term benefits for five elements of metabolic syndrome (a risk factor for heart disease): waist circumference, triglyceride levels, blood pressure, HDL cholesterol, and fasting blood sugar.

Cutting out complete food categories, as the paleo diet does, leads to an extremely restricted diet that is difficult to maintain over time. On the autoimmune paleo diet, you may miss out on important nutrients by eliminating whole food categories. Consider dairy items such as cheese, yogurt, and milk. These can be rich in calcium and vitamin D, which are both important for bone health.

People who adopted an autoimmune paleo diet only got half of the required calcium dose. As a result, nutritional shortages are one of the autoimmune paleo diet's health risks.

Autoimmune paleo dieters must be cautious about the sorts of meat they consume. Red meat has a lot of saturated fat, which can raise your cholesterol and increase your risk of heart disease and stroke. Red meat should be taken in moderation, no more than twice a week.

References:

1. MayoClinic. *"Paleo Diet: What Is It And Why Is It So Popular?"* Retrieved from Mayoclinic.org: https://www.mayoclinic.org/healthy-lifestyle/nutrition-and-healthy-eating/in-depth/paleo-diet/art-20111182

2. Lisa. *"Is The Autoimmune Paleo Diet Legit?"* Retrieved from USnews.com: https://health.usnews.com/health-news/health-wellness/articles/2015/01/16/is-the-autoimmune-paleo-diet-legit

3. Carol. *"Does The Autoimmune Protocol Diet Help Rheumatoid Arthritis?"* Retrieved from Everydayhealth.com: https://www.everydayhealth.com/rheumatoid-arthritis/auto-immune-protocol-diet-aip-diet-ra/

4. Davis, U. *"Paleo Diet: What It Is And Why It's Not For Everyone"*. Retrieved from Ucdavis.edu: https://health.ucdavis.edu/blog/good-food/paleo-diet-what-it-is-and-why-its-not-for-everyone/2022/04

5. Gaurree. *"Efficacy Of The Autoimmune Protocol Diet For In-flammatory Bowel Disease"*. Retrieved from Nih.gov: https://www.ncbi.nlm.nih.gov/pmc/articles/PMC5647120/

Chapter 14

A HEALTHY APPROACH TO
REDUCING INFLAMMATION

Inflammation protects you from bacterial and viral infections by releasing chemicals from white blood cells.

Inflammation is the response of the immune system to perceived injury or infection. When damage has occurred, inflammation is beneficial. An army of white blood cells attacks the infection and promotes healing. When infected by a virus or infection, the body responds similarly.

However, this immunological response can occasionally malfunction. It can be triggered by pollutants, stress, obesity, and autoimmune illnesses. Frequently, inflammation remains instead of fading and returning to normal. Chronic inflammation may result in heart disease, arthritis, depression, Alzheimer's disease, and cancer.

Avoid red meat, processed carbohydrates (such as white bread and muffins), fried foods, and sugary beverages to prevent chronic inflammation. Choose leafy greens, almonds, seafood high in fat, and olive oil. Focus on exercise, rest, and stress management.

In many diseases, including arthritis, the immune system initiates inflammation without infection. In autoimmune diseases, the immune system assaults and damages normal tissues.

Negative Impacts of Inflammation:

- **It can affect the digestive tract:**

Denning states that many immune cells congregate near the intestines. The majority of the time, these immune cells overlook the billions of good gut flora. "However, this tolerance appears to be broken in some individuals," adds Denning. "Their immune cells begin to respond to the bacteria, causing chronic inflammation."

- **It can cause joint damage:**

When inflammation arises in the joints, severe damage can result. Rheumatoid arthritis (RA) is a joint-damaging autoimmune disorder that appears to have a genetic component. Still, it is also associated with smoking, a deficiency in vitamin D, and other risk factors. According to a 2013 Yale University study, a salty diet may contribute to rheumatoid arthritis (RA) development.

- **It is associated with heart disease:**

Even the inside of blood vessels can become inflamed if they have been harmed or compromised. Chronic inflammation can be caused by the buildup of fatty plaque in the arteries. The fatty plaques attract white blood cells, become larger, and can induce a heart attack by forming blood clots. According to a study published in The Lancet in 2012, interleukin-6 (IL-6) may significantly influence.

Obesity and improper eating promote inflammation in the body. Still, even healthy people with chronic inflammation due to an autoimmune disorder, such as rheumatoid arthritis, psoriasis, or celiac disease, tend to have a higher risk of heart disease, regardless of their weight or eating habits.

- **It is associated with greater cancer risk:**

With so much commotion surrounding potential causes of cancer (underwire bras, really?), it is difficult to identify the real dangers. The good news is that there are not many specific food types associated with cancer.

- **It may damage your sleep**

Insufficiency in sleep is associated with a variety of health issues, including depression and cardiovascular disease. Ensure that you fall asleep soon so that you can obtain a restful night's sleep. Watch this video to learn six basic methods for combating insomnia.

- **It is harmful to the lungs:**

Inflammation in the lungs can lead to fluid collection and airway constriction, making breathing harder. Lung inflammation is characteristic of infections, asthma, and chronic obstructive pulmonary disease (COPD), including emphysema and chronic bronchitis.

- **It harms gums:**

Inflammation can also wreak havoc on the mouth in the form of periodontitis, a bacterial accumulation-induced chronic inflammation of the gums. This condition causes gum recession and weakening or injury to the skeletal bone surrounding the teeth.

- **It deteriorates bone:**

According to a review article published in the Journal of Endocrinology in 2009, inflammation throughout the body can inhibit bone formation and even cause increased bone loss. Researchers hypothesize that inflammatory indicators in the blood impede "remodeling" — the continuous process by which old, broken bone fragments are replaced with new ones.

- **It impacts the skin:**

The effects of inflammation are not limited to internal manifestations; they can also manifest on the skin. Psoriasis, for instance, is an inflammatory illness that occurs when the immune system promotes excessive skin cell growth. Since obesity leads to inflammation, a 2013 study published in JAMA Dermatology suggested that weight loss could help psoriasis patients find relief.

What are the medical approaches to reducing inflammation and what kind of side effects do they have?

Not all cases of inflammation require therapy. In a matter of days, rest, ice, and proper wound care typically alleviate the pain associated with acute inflammation.

If you suffer from persistent inflammation, your doctor may recommend:

1. Supplements: Certain vitamins (vitamin A, vitamin C, vitamin D) and supplements (zinc) may reduce inflammation and promote repair. For instance, your doctor may recommend a fish oil supplement or vitamin (s). Alternatively, you may take anti-inflammatory spices such as turmeric, Ginger, or garlic.

Side-effects:

You are more likely to experience adverse effects from dietary supplements if you take them in large dosages, substitute them for prescribed medications, or take multiple supplements. Certain nutritional supplements can raise the risk of bleeding or alter the reaction to anesthetic if taken prior to surgery. Some supplements can interact with certain medications in ways that can be problematic. Here are few instances:

- Vitamin K can inhibit the anticoagulant drug warfarin's ability to prevent blood from clotting.
- St. John's wort can accelerate the breakdown of several medications and diminish their efficacy (including some antidepressants, birth control pills, heart medications, anti-HIV medications, and transplant drugs).
- Antioxidant supplements, such as vitamins C and E, may diminish the efficacy of certain cancer chemotherapy regimens.

2. Nonsteroidal anti-inflammatory drugs (NSAIDs): These over-the-counter medications lower inflammation. Your physician may prescribe ibuprofen (Advil®), aspirin (Bayer®), or naproxen (Aleve®).

Side-effects:

- Indigestion, including abdominal pain, nausea, and diarrhea.
- Stomach ulcers can lead to internal bleeding and anaemia; additional medication to protect the stomach may be administered to lessen this risk.
- Headaches, sleepiness, vertigo, and allergic responses are common side effects.

3. **Steroid injections:** Corticosteroid shots reduce inflammation at the a specific joint or muscle. If you have rheumatoid arthritis that affects your back, your healthcare professional may administer a steroid injection into your spine. No more than 3 to 4 steroid injections should be administered annually to the same body part.

Side-effects:

- Pain at the injection site, ranging from mild to severe, is commonly referred to as a cortisone or steroid flare.
- localized bruising at the injection site.
- The face flushed for several hours.
- Skin that is thin or pallid around the injection site.
- insomnia.

How can inflammation be prevented?

By maintaining healthy lifestyle behaviors, you can reduce your risk of chronic inflammation. Several of these practices include:

- Obtaining and keeping a healthy weight.
- Avoiding or quitting smoking.
- At least three to five times a week of exercise (daily exercise is best).
- Limiting alcohol consumption (maximum 2 ounces per day).
- Utilizing healthy stress management techniques such as meditation and journaling.

Why is the Cox 2 pathway so important to address, and why do standard pharmaceutical approaches to reducing inflammation often involve activating the Cox-1 pathway, which can lead to

complications associated with the stomach, kidneys, and the heart?

In the 1990s, it was discovered that the cyclooxygenase enzyme exists in two forms: COX-1 and COX-2.3. This factor is responsible for in-flammation. COX-1 is recognized to be found in the majority of our body's tissues. COX-1 supports the proper lining of the stomach and intestines in the gastrointestinal tract, protecting the stomach from di-gestive fluids. Additionally, the enzyme has a role in kidney and plate-let function.

COX-2, on the other hand, is predominantly prevalent at inflammatory locations. Both COX-1 and COX-2 create the prostaglandins that con-tribute to pain, fever, and inflammation. However, because COX-1's major function protects the stomach and intestines and contributes to blood clotting, medicines that block COX-1 might have undesirable side effects.

Side-effects:

- **GI Effects:**

COX inhibitors can induce discomfort in the upper and lower gastro-intestinal tracts and bleeding and perforation. The elderly, people with peptic ulcers, and those using steroids or blood thinners are at danger. NSAIDs should not be taken.

Common upper GI symptoms:

Dyspepsia, heartburn, and nausea are gastrointestinal (GI) side effects. Possible mucosal damage and ulceration Ulcers that bleed necessitate endoscopic treatment and proton pump inhibitors.

75% of NSAID users report gastrointestinal issues.

Ulcers, bleeding, and obstructions may develop. Treatments include discontinuing medication and endoscopic procedures.

In extreme situations, laparotomy and intestinal resection are required. Celecoxib and proton pump inhibitors reduce gastrointestinal adverse effects. Proton pump inhibitors do not affect lower GI adverse effects and are exclusively safe for the stomach. PPIs are associated with damage to the small intestine.

H. pylori raises the risk of peptic ulcer disease among NSAID users. Before taking NSAIDs, eradicating H. pylori helps avoid upper gastrointestinal ulcers.

- **CV Outcome:**

Cox inhibitors other than aspirin increase the risk of MI, CVD, and stroke. Patients with cardiovascular disease are at a greater risk. The overall risk is lower than that of GI.

In 2015, the FDA revised the warning label for NSAIDs. The risk of myocardial infarction peaks seven days after NSAID use. Celecoxib therapy for 30 days is required. This risk persisted for 3 weeks following nonselective NSAIDs and 3.5 months following celecoxib.

Cox inhibitors are associated with a 1% to 5% renal risk.

COX inhibitors, NSAIDs, and COX-2 NSAIDs are all toxic to the kidneys. The renal afferent arterioles are constrained. In the case of hypovolemia or renal illness, caution is suggested. The kidney expresses the inducible COX-2 gene constitutively.

- **Hematology:**

The thromboxane A2 inhibits platelets. Because COX is irreversibly inhibited, platelet inhibition persists for 7–10 days after aspirin withdrawal. Alcohol, anticoagulants, and liver disease all induce bleeding.

Platelets prevent haemorrhage. NSAIDs suppress platelets in a dose- and half-life-dependent manner. Nonselective NSAIDs reduce aspirin's anti-aggregate effect, hence increasing cardiovascular risk. COX-2 inhibitors unalter the antiplatelet action of aspirin.

- **Malignancy:**

COX inhibitors are anti-cancer agents. In a variety of ways, aspirin suppresses colon cancer. Patients at risk for cardiovascular disease should be selected.

Aspirin and nonsteroidal anti-inflammatory drugs (NSAIDs) have also been investigated for prostate cancer, and COX inhibitors may reduce risk, although there are no clear guidelines or explanations. Long-term effects must be weighed equally. COX inhibitors improve survival in ovarian cancer patients.

- **Sensitivity:**

NSAIDs frequently result in hypersensitivity. NSAIDs cause multiple complex hypersensitivity responses. Multiple pathways contribute to hypersensitivity. They can be caused by selective responders or nonsteroidal anti-inflammatory drugs (cross intolerant).

Some of the symptoms include urticaria, rhinitis, asthma, angioedema, bullous or desquamating lesions, DRESS syndrome, and toxic epidermal necrolysis. The responses include bile duct syndrome, meningitis, and vasculitis—IgE, T-cell, suppression of prostaglandin, or unknown.

Common hypersensitivity reaction: respiratory disease worsened by NSAIDs. There is a role for eosinophils and other mediators. Rhinitis, polyps, sinusitis, and asthma are caused by persistent inflammation.

Top natural Anti-inflammatory herbs and supplements that our clinic recommends:

Some natural supplements may aid in the battle against inflammation, although not all nutrients are effective against all forms of inflammation.

This article describes some of the most effective anti-inflammatory supplements that individuals may wish to take, depending on the source of their inflammation.

- **Omega-3 fatty acids:**

Omega-3 fatty acids may aid in the battle against vascular inflammation.

These nutrients may aid in combating various inflammatory conditions, including vascular inflammation. Vascular inflammation is a substantial cardiovascular disease and heart attack risk factor.

- **Curcumin:**

Curcumin, the key element in turmeric, is a plant belonging to the ginger family. Studies on animals suggest that it may help reduce inflammation to accelerate wound healing and perhaps lessen cancer risk.

A 2011 study indicated that curcumin might help reduce inflammation caused by metabolic problems associated with obesity. Curcumin modified many inflammatory pathways, hence decreasing insulin resistance, hyperglycemia, and hyperlipidemia.

- **S-adenosylmethionine:**

S-adenosylmethionine (SAM-e) is a chemical produced by the body. It is crucial to the epigenetic control of genes.

As inflammation may play a role in depression, osteoarthritis, and some liver disorders, SAM-e is sometimes used to treat their symptoms.

A small number of scientific investigations suggest that SAM-e may help alleviate the pain and inflammation associated with various types of arthritis – sometimes as effectively as nonsteroidal anti-inflammatory drugs (NSAIDs).

- **Zinc:**

According to research, zinc reduces oxidative stress in older persons.

According to some studies, zinc is a strong anti-inflammatory that may boost the immune system and lower various inflammatory indicators.

Zinc lowered inflammation and oxidative stress in older persons, according to a 2014 study. Oxidative stress may increase the risk of various diseases, including cancer, by inducing inflammation.

In addition, zinc lowered the incidence of infections by 66%.

Arthritis is more prevalent in zinc-deficient individuals, suggesting a connection between zinc deficiency, inflammation, and pain.

- **Green tea:**

Doctors have long suspected that green tea may be anti-inflammatory because locations with more green tea consumption had lower rates of inflammation-related diseases.

According to research, green tea may suppress the development of some pro-inflammatory substances. It may also help reduce cartilage loss, so lowering arthritic symptoms.

- **Frankincense:**

Frankincense can reduce inflammation and pain.

Additionally, it may prevent cartilage loss and restore autoimmune symptoms. It is a vitamin that may relieve osteoarthritis pain within five days.

The typical daily dosage is 300–500 mg of an extract containing 30–40 percent boswellic acids, taken in doses of two to three times each day.

- **Capsaicin:**

Capsaicin is the component responsible for the spiciness of hot peppers. Substance P, an essential component of capsaicin, may lower the body's sensitivity to the transmission of pain.

Some study indicates that capsaicin may alleviate nerve and muscle discomfort.

Several manufacturers sell lotions containing capsaicin that can be directly applied to sore locations.

- **Cat's claw:**

Cat's claw derives from different Uncaria plants, including Uncaria tomentosa and Uncaria guianensis.

According to research, cat's claw may alleviate several types of inflammation. It is compelling at inhibiting TNF-alpha, an inflammatory substance in the body.

What is Boswellia and how can it reduce inflammation?

Boswellia, commonly referred to as Indian frankincense, is a botanical extract derived from the Boswellia serrata tree.

In traditional Asian and African medicine, resin prepared from Boswellia extract has been employed for generations. It is believed to cure chronic inflammatory diseases in addition to a variety of other disorders. Boswellia can be obtained as a resin, a tablet, or a lotion.

Boswellic acid can prevent the development of leukotrienes in the body, according to some research. Leukotrienes have been discovered as chemicals that cause inflammation. They could provoke asthma symptoms.

Boswellia resin contains four acids that contribute to the herb's anti-inflammatory capabilities. These acids inhibit 5-lipoxygenase (5-LO), the enzyme responsible for leukotriene production. It is believed that acetyl-11-keto—boswellic acid (AKBA) is the most potent of the four boswellic acids. However, other research suggests that the herb's anti-inflammatory benefits are due to other boswellic acids.

Boswellia products are often graded based on their boswellic acid concentration.

Boswellia may be beneficial in treating inflammatory bowel illnesses such as Crohn's disease and ulcerative colitis due to the herb's anti-inflammatory effects (UC).

In a 2001 study, H15, a unique Boswellia extract, as compared to the anti-inflammatory prescription medication mesalamine (Apriso, Asacol HD). It demonstrated that Boswellia extract may be helpful in treating Crohn's disease.

According to Reliable Source, the plant may also help treat UC. Just now we are beginning to comprehend how the anti-inflammatory and immune-balancing actions of Boswellia can improve the health of an inflamed colon.

What is Ginger and how can it reduce inflammation?

Ginger is a flowering plant indigenous to numerous Asian, West African, and Caribbean regions. It is closely related to cardamom and turmeric. It has been utilized for millennia in traditional Asian medicine.

It may assist with a variety of health concerns, including cardiovascular illness, motion sickness, osteoarthritis, and rheumatoid arthritis.

Due to its antioxidant and anti-inflammatory qualities, Ginger may help prevent and treat arthritis.

There are about 1,300 varieties of ginger plants, and they contain a variety of nutrients, including:

- Vitamin C and vitamin B6 the minerals magnesium, potassium, and copper.
- Phytonutrients and polyphenols such as gingerols, shogaols, and paradols.
- Gingerol and paradols are both anti-inflammatory and possess antioxidant effects. Antioxidants eliminate free radicals, which can cause cell damage and inflammation in the body.

When the immune system attempts to avoid damage to the body, inflammation ensues. It might cause discomfort and edoema.

Symptoms of osteoarthritis, rheumatoid arthritis, and other kinds of arthritis include pain and inflammation. Consuming antioxidants prevent the cellular damage associated with these illnesses.

As a treatment for arthritis, nonsteroidal anti-inflammatory medications (NSAIDs) are frequently prescribed. Ginger may be an alternative treatment option for certain symptoms.

What is Alpha-Lipoic Acid and how can it reduce inflammation?

Alpha-lipoic acid is an organic compound found in all human cells.

It is produced within the mitochondrion, also known as the cell's powerhouse, where it assists enzymes in converting nutrients into energy.

Additionally, it possesses potent antioxidant effects.

Alpha-lipoic acid is soluble in both water and fat, allowing it to function in every cell and tissue of the body. Meanwhile, the majority of other antioxidants are either water- or fat-soluble. Vitamin C, for instance, is only water-soluble, whereas vitamin E is only fat-soluble.

Several benefits have been associated with the antioxidant characteristics of alpha-lipoic acid, including lower blood sugar levels, reduced inflammation, slower skin ageing, and enhanced neurological function.

Humans produce small amounts of alpha-lipoic acid. Consequently, many individuals turn to specific foods or supplements to improve their consumption.

However, plant foods such as broccoli, tomatoes, spinach, and Brussels sprouts also contain alpha-lipoic acid.

Several diseases, including cancer and diabetes, are connected to chronic inflammation. Alpha-lipoic acid has been proven to reduce a number of inflammatory indicators.

Alpha-lipoic acid significantly decreased levels of the inflammatory marker C-reactive protein (CRP) in people with high levels of CRP, according to a meta-analysis of 11 trials.

What is Celery Seed Extract and how can it reduce inflammation?

Popular as a vegetable, celery comprises more than just the stalk. Celery seeds are uncommon yet pleasant and healthful nonetheless.

They are tiny, light-brown, and emit an earthy odor. Their flavor is harsh and warm.

Celery seeds have been used in Eastern medicine for thousands of years to cure bronchitis, skin diseases, and the flu.

Today, celery seeds are most frequently employed as a seasoning. However, they are also available as an extract or pill supplement.

Although small in size, celery seeds are highly nutritious and offer numerous health advantages.

Many diseases, including arthritis and osteoporosis, have been related to chronic inflammation. There are roughly 25 anti-inflammatory chemicals in celery and celery seeds that offer protection against inflammation in the body.

What is Collagen, and how can it reduce inflammation?

Collagen is recognized as the body's most abundant protein. It may be found in skin, bones, cartilage, tendons, and teeth and is the primary component of the body's connective tissues. Collagen fibres maintain the majority of the body's tissues and may be found both inside and outside of cells.

Collagen II alleviates arthritic pain. Chicken in general. Unproven: It induces the production of anti-inflammatory chemicals in the body. With chondroitin and glucosamine, chicken collagen may help mend cartilage.

Chondroitin and glucosamine supplements for OA are not supported by solid evidence.

- **Osteoarthritis:**

Osteoarthritis affects about 32,5 million persons.

Deteriorated cartilage is the reason. Inconclusive is the research on collagen supplements for osteoarthritis.

The effects of acetaminophen and Collagen on knee osteoarthritis pain, function, and quality of life were enhanced. The research had 39 participants.

Collagen hydrolysate and undenatured Collagen may aid in treating osteoarthritis, but more study is required.

- **Rheumatoid Arthritis:**

When the immune system targets healthy cells, the hands, wrists, and knees experience severe swelling. In RA, inflammation can cause joint tissue damage. Collagen supplementation in RA has variable outcomes.

Oral UC-II and denatured Collagen may alleviate OA discomfort.

Few long-term research indicates the advantages of Collagen. According to preclinical and clinical studies, oral Collagen is advantageous for RA.

What is a natural eggshell membrane, and how can it reduce inflammation?

Calcium carbonate ($CaCO3$) crystals compose almost the whole of eggshell. This membrane is semipermeable, so air and water may enter through its holes. Additionally, the shell contains a thin exterior layer known as the bloom or cuticle, which keeps out germs and dust.

Natural Eggshell Membrane (NEM®) is a potential new effective and safe therapeutic alternative for treating joint and connective tissue (JCT)-related pain and stiffness. Supplementation with 500 mg of NEM® once daily dramatically decreased pain fast (within seven days) and constantly (30 days). In addition, a quick responder analysis revealed clinically significant outcomes, suggesting that a substantial percentage of treated patients may benefit significantly from NEM® supplementation.

Chapter 15

HOW L-ARGININE CAN IMPROVE YOUR NEUROPATHY

What Is L-Arginine?

It seems as though every time you turn around, you are faced with someone talking about L-arginine benefits. While many trends seem to come and go in the health field, this is one that is here to stay. This is because this is not a trend and it is not something unnatural. Anytime you can give your body more of what it should be getting in your diet; it's beneficial. This is why people take vitamins, especially those that barely find the time to eat anything that doesn't come out of a bag, box or can. People are trying it and experiencing for themselves how great they feel! So, what is L-arginine?

L-arginine is an amino acid that helps make proteins. It also becomes the gas Nitric Oxide (NO) in the body. L-Arginine is a conditionally essential amino acid found in the diet. It is a dietary supplement used mostly by athletic people because it is the amino acid that directly produces nitric oxide via the nitric oxide synthase enzymes.

Nitric Oxide is important for erectile function because it helps blood vessels relax so that more oxygen-rich blood can circulate through your arteries. Healthy blood flow to the arteries of the penis is essential for normal erectile function.

L-Arginine is a particular amino acid in the body that is going to be involved with a number of different body functions. First, it is going to play a vital role in wound healing, so for anyone suffering from injuries, it can assist with this. In addition to that, L-arginine is also going to be useful for helping the kidneys remove excess waste products from the body, helping you function and feel that much better on a day to day basis. Furthermore, L-arginine is also corrected with maintaining a strong immune system and proper hormonal function - both of which are also vital for optimizing your health state.

While you will take in L-arginine from some of the foods that you eat on a daily basis, often you won't get concentrated enough levels to see real benefits occurring. That's where supplementation comes in helpful.

What Are The Benefits Of L-Arginine?

If you are wondering what exactly L arginine is and what are its benefits to the human body, then you will be glad to know that you are reading the benefits of L arginine. L arginine is an amino acid which helps in the production of proteins in the human body. The human body is able to maintain the needed amounts of arginine by its own, but during situations like severe burns, infections, injuries, and aging, the supply gets reduced. When the human body undergoes such situations, it is only wise that you increase your intake of arginine.

In the body, the amino acid arginine changes into nitric oxide (NO). Nitric oxide is a powerful neurotransmitter that helps blood vessels relax and also improves circulation. Some evidence shows that arginine may help improve blood flow in the arteries of the heart. Since arginine may help arteries to relax and enhance blood flow, it may also help with erectile dysfunction.

There are other potential health benefits of L arginine to the human body which include the following:

Brain Function: Oxygen flow to the brain decreases with age, as does the production of l-arginine and nitric oxide. With this decrease in oxygen flow to the brain comes decreased brain function. L-arginine benefits healthy blood flow to areas of the brain, and because the cells in the brain are continually working, optimal brain function requires optimal blood flow.

Immune System: While the heart benefits of L-arginine are numerous, L-arginine has also been scientifically proven to improve the body's immune system by increasing the size and strength of the thymus. The thymus is the endocrine system gland the produces T cells, also known as 'fighting cells,' responsible for fighting off infection.

Erectile Dysfunction: The many benefits of L-arginine are pretty well known, especially its positive effect on erectile dysfunction. Many studies have gone to show improvement in sexual function for men with erectile dysfunction who take L-arginine supplements. L-arginine's ability to increase blood flow and relax the artery walls also makes it very effective at relaxing the smooth muscle within the penis, improving blood flow and decreasing symptoms of erectile dysfunction.

High blood pressure: There is early evidence that taking L-arginine by mouth can reduce blood pressure in healthy people, people with high blood pressure, and people with slightly high blood pressure with or without diabetes.

Heart Failure: Taking L-arginine by mouth, together with conventional treatment, seems to improve kidney function in people with heart failure. However, it might not improve the ability to exercise, quality of life, or blood circulation. L-arginine should not be used in place of conventional treatment.

Critical Illness (trauma): Research shows that taking L-arginine by mouth with glutamine, nucleotides, and omega-3 fatty acids reduce the recovery time, the need for help with breathing, and risk of infections in people who are critically ill. However, it does not reduce the risk of death.

Diabetes: Taking L-arginine by mouth seems to improve blood sugar control in people with existing diabetes. However, it is unclear if arginine helps prevent people with pre-diabetes from developing diabetes.

Exercise performance: There is inconsistent evidence about the effects of L-arginine on exercise performance. Some evidence shows that taking 6 grams of L-arginine in a drink increases exercise time until becoming tired. Also taking arginine with grape seed extract appears to improve working ability in men and decreases their tiredness. However, taking arginine 6 grams once does not affect strength during exercise.

Sickle-cell disease: Early research suggests that taking L-arginine for 5 days might be useful for people with sickle cell disease who have high blood pressure in the lungs.

Stress: Some early research suggests that taking a combination of L-lysine and L-arginine for up to 10 days reduces stress and anxiety in healthy people and those prone to stress.

L-Arginine Supplementation Increases Stamina: Studies have shown that L-arginine can decrease the amount of oxygen needed by muscles during exercise. This increases the amount of time a muscle can be exercised before it is exhausted.

What Is The Science Behind L-Arginine?

L Arginine is a conditionally essential amino acid that is involved in protein synthesis, the detoxification of ammonia, and its conversion to glucose as well as being catabolized to produce energy. It is a vitally important amino acid that has been studied for more than half a century. Amino acids are the building blocks of protein, and protein is the building block of all living cells. The greatest portion of human body weight, after water, is protein.

L-arginine is a chemical building block called "an amino acid." It is obtained from the diet and is necessary for the body to make proteins. L-arginine is found in red meat, poultry, fish, and dairy products. It can also be made in a laboratory and used as medicine. The study of amino acids is making a major contribution to the understanding of many diseases. Amino acid therapies have been used successfully to prevent aging, prevent heart disease, enhance memory, eliminate depression, control stress, improve sleep, relieve arthritis, reduce herpes, arrest alcoholism, manage allergies, and much more.

L-arginine is converted in the body into a chemical called nitric oxide. Nitric oxide causes blood vessels to open wider for improved blood flow. L-arginine also stimulates the release of growth hormone, insulin, and other substances in the body. L-Arginine can help boost the production of nitric oxide in the body, and nitric oxide will then help relax blood vessels and improve circulation. For anyone with issues related to high blood pressure or poor circulation then, this supplement can provide some relief. Because this amino does this, it's a powerful way to improve symptoms of clogged arteries, angina, as well as coronary artery disease.

In addition to boosting heart health, another of the L-Arginine benefits to know is that it can also help to lower your risk of stroke as well. Once again, this is due to enhanced blood circulation. Males who are suffering from any erectile dysfunction may also have vested interest in the L-Arginine benefits they can see as supplementing with this amino acid may help to improve sexual performance reduce this problem.

While most people will respond relatively well to L-arginine supplementation, it's not without side effects. This supplement can cause issues such as indigestion, nausea, headaches, bloating, diarrhea, as well as low blood pressure in some people.

Furthermore, it's recommended that those who suffer from diabetes should stay away from L-arginine as well as anyone who is pregnant or nursing.

How Can L-Arginine Help Someone With Neuropathy?

Neuropathy, also known as peripheral neuropathy, is certainly one of the most common chronic diseases in the United States. Peripheral neuropathy is a disorder of the peripheral nerves - the autonomic, sensory and motor nerves that connect the spinal cord to muscles, skin and the internal organs. It normally affects the feet and hands of the afflicted person - with varying results such as weakness, tingling, pain and numbness in these extremities. Neuropathy is "nerve damage" that can be compared to the body's electrical wiring system breaking down - it disrupts the body's ability to communicate with the skin, joints, muscles or internal organs.

Peripheral Neuropathy gradually consumes your focus and eventually the doctors end up prescribing painful tests of the musculature of the limbs and then advocate for medications to calm the nerve endings that tear you out of your sleep with cramps and pain and leave you feeling exhausted at the end of the night; knowing that once again your peace and calm have been wracked by an unseen monster in your peripheral limbs.

But...there is an answer – L-arginine has been shown in many case studies to provide a way to escalate the circulation to the peripheral limbs that in turn, resolve the issue of circulation and blood flow through the creation of Nitric Oxide. This causes the muscles to relax, restoring elasticity to arteries that have become rigid from age and plaque buildup. In turn, it increases the artery's ability to move blood and the nutrients that it carries much more efficiently than before.

This most basic improvement to the circulatory system alone allows the blood to deliver far more of the daily nutrients that our bodies need, far more efficiently and easily. L-Arginine helps supply nitric oxide for wound healing and improves circulation, which can be of great benefit in diabetic peripheral neuropathy.

What Exactly Does L-Arginine Do With Blood Flow?

L-arginine is an amino acid that your body converts to nitric oxide, which boosts circulation and blood flow by dilating your blood vessels. One of the biggest benefits of taking L-arginine is its ability to improve blood flow and circulation. In the body, it is converted into nitric oxide, which causes blood vessels to open wider. L-arginine releases nitric oxide in the blood. Nitric oxide acts to widen blood vessels in the bloodstream, which may help aid certain circulatory conditions.

Nitric oxide improves circulation by dialing blood vessels, so when people don't have enough in their arteries their risk for heart disease is higher. NO keeps your blood pressure level within a normal range by signaling blood vessel muscles to relax, expand and let blood through, while also preventing clots and plaque from forming. Research suggests that as someone ages, his or her ability to produce enough NO in the artery linings decreases, but luckily obtaining more L-arginine — either through supplemental arginine or dietary arginine — can enhance nitric oxide capabilities and correct impaired endothelial function.

By improving blood flow in the body, some proponents claim that L-arginine may help heart conditions, such as chest pain (angina), high blood pressure, leg cramping and weakness due to obstructed arteries (a condition known as intermittent claudication), and erectile dysfunction (ED).

L-arginine is considered somewhat essential because it's highly important for many functions yet usually present in low quantities, especially as someone gets older. This has multiple benefits, including improving immune function, fertility, detoxification, and brain power. Another important aspect of L-arginine is that it stimulates the production of certain hormones, especially beneficial growth hormones and insulin that help usher glucose into cells to be used for growth and energy output. This is one of the reasons it's believed to enhance physical performance, stamina and strength.

How Long Does It Take To See Results With L-Arginine?

L-arginine is a semi-essential amino acid. This means that the body normally produces adequate amounts of it. However, certain people such as infants and people with particular health conditions do not produce enough of it. They, therefore, need to get an adequate amount of l-arginine either through foods or supplements. L-arginine is commonly found in foods such as dairy products, meats, seafood, grains, nuts, seeds, peas, and beans.

Doses vary widely, depending on the conditions being treated, most of which lack established therapeutic dose ranges. Studies have involved doses ranging from 700 milligrams to 20 grams given from one to four times a day. Individuals who self-treat with L-arginine supplements may combine it with other supplements.

Also, how much you take often depends on the reason you're taking l-arginine in the first place. People with high blood pressure typically take between 5,000mg to 10,000mg a day. If you're taking L-arginine to increase your energy levels, support your immune system or just to improve your overall health, somewhere between 4,000 to 6,000mg is generally enough to make a difference.

If you take too much l-arginine, your blood pressure could drop too low, or your electrolytes could get off balance. This will most likely happen if you take way more than what your body needs, but it is better to start smaller and work from there.

So how long does it take for L- Arginine to work in the body? How long it take L arginine to turn into nitric oxide when it enters the body, depend on the person. Because I know everybody has a body that works differently than others. While some people may see results as early as the next day, the suggested time to take is about two weeks. After two or three weeks, the effects of l-arginine on blood pressure and a difference in workout endurance should be evident.

What Does L-Arginine Do To The Cardiovascular System?

The human cardiovascular system is an organ system that conveys blood through vessels to and from all parts of the body, carrying nutrients and oxygen to tissues and removing carbon dioxide and other wastes. It is a closed tubular system in which the blood is propelled by a muscular heart. Two circuits, the pulmonary and the systemic, consist of arterial, capillary, and venous components. The cardiovascular system is an organ system that permits blood to circulate and transport nutrients (such as amino acids and electrolytes), oxygen, carbon dioxide, hormones, and blood cells to and from the cells in the body to provide nourishment and help in fighting diseases, stabilize temperature and pH, and maintain homeostasis.

The amino acid, L-Arginine plays a vital role in the cardiovascular system. A recent study shows that L-Arginine is the only substrate for the production of Nitric Oxide (NO), from which L-Arginine develops its effects on the cardiovascular system. As a free radical, NO is synthesized in all mammalian cells by L-Arginine with the activity of nitric oxide synthase.

In states of hypertension, diabetes, hypercholesterolemia and vascular inflammation, a disorder occurs in the metabolic pathway of the synthesis of NO from L-Arginine which all together bring alterations of blood vessels. Experimental results obtained on animals, as well as clinical studies, show that L-Arginine affects thrombocytes, on the process of coagulation and the fibrolytic system.

What Does L-Arginine Do To The Blood Flow?

L-Arginine is a vasodilator, that is, it dilates the blood vessels, allowing more blood to pass through at once for improved blood flow. The enhanced blood flow will help carry nutrients to your muscles. Arginine stimulates protein production and also stimulates the release of insulin (which is an important nutrient to shuttle protein into the muscles).

L-arginine is an amino acid that helps make proteins. It also becomes the gas Nitric Oxide (NO) in the body. NO is important for erectile function because it helps blood vessels relax so that more oxygen-rich blood can circulate through your arteries. Healthy blood flow to the arteries of the penis is essential for normal erectile function.

L-arginine is converted in the body into a chemical called nitric oxide. Nitric oxide causes blood vessels to open wider for improved blood flow. By improving blood flow in the body, some proponents claim that L-arginine may help heart conditions, such as chest pain (angina), high blood pressure, leg cramping and weakness due to obstructed arteries (a condition known as intermittent claudication), and Erectile Dysfunction (ED).

More specifically, L-Arginine restores production of nitric oxide to the body, a key element in improving blood flow. When blood is able to flow more freely through the blood vessels, you feel more energetic because your heart does not have to work as hard to pump blood throughout the body. You are also better able to fight off disease because your blood is better able to provide infection sites with healthy blood cells.

Increasing your body's defenses does not only provide benefits against common illnesses but by increasing your body's defenses, you can also increase your ability to ward off more traumatic illnesses such as cardiovascular disease. A more free flow of blood means that cramping due to poor blood flow as well as fatigue is improved, if not avoided. The heart then does not have to work as hard to pump blood to the rest of the body. A healthy heart allows individuals with the opportunities to lead longer and healthier lives.

Chapter 16

WHAT IS L-CITRULLINE?

L-citrulline is a substance that is a non-essential amino acid. It is actively found and changed in our kidneys into another amino acid, called L-arginine and a chemical known as nitric oxide. Amazingly important for the heart and blood vessel health, these compounds play an active role in boosting the immune system.

L-Citrulline is an amino acid that is produced naturally by your body. It is found in some foods like watermelons and is also produced naturally by the body. For those of you unfamiliar with amino acids, they are the building blocks of protein in your body, which are responsible for numerous beneficial functions. Our body actually converts L-Citrulline to that other confusing word below (L-Arginine). Ultimately that conversion leads to the production of nitric oxide.

L-citrulline is used for Alzheimer's disease, dementia, fatigue, muscle weakness, sickle cell disease, erectile dysfunction, high blood pressure, and diabetes. It is used for heart disease, bodybuilding, increasing energy, and for improving athletic performance.

The main effect of L-citrulline is to produce nitric oxide within the body, which is a substance that helps the arteries relax and work better. This significantly improves the blood flow throughout the body and may be helpful for either treating or preventing many diseases.

Most importantly, L-citrulline plays a vital role in the urea cycle, a process where the body eliminates toxic byproducts that happen from digesting protein and generation cellular energy. These waste products are converted into a substance called urea, expelled from the body through the urine and sweat.

Lastly, L-Citrulline is most prominent in watermelons, but it can also be found in lower dosages in foods like; walnuts, meat, fish, eggs, milk, and legumes.

What Are The Benefits Of L-Citrulline?

The role of L-Citrulline when it is used as a supplement is to improve blood flow in the body by converting to L-Arginine. The increase in L-Arginine provides benefits to the heart that are the result of a more easily flowing bloodstream that is due to the effects that L-Arginine has on nitric oxide. Nitric oxide is a compound that relaxes blood vessels. The more relaxed the blood vessels are, the better they can handle the flow of blood that runs through them. The benefits of L-Citrulline and L-Arginine are intertwined. The result of improved production of nitric oxide and better blood flow helps to ease physical fatigue (and some would argue mental fatigue also) as well as improve sexual function in both men and women (although the change is most dramatically seen by men who had previously been suffering from impotence before beginning an L-Citrulline/L-Arginine dietary supplement).

As you can see anything that can aid the body in increasing amino acids and nitric oxide is going to do wonders to how your body functions and thus how you feel every day. The benefits of using L-Citrulline as a dietary supplement are impressive, diverse and natural. These benefits are waiting to be had by the great majority of us (except those individuals currently on medication or receiving treatment that may not allow for the safe use of L-Citrulline or similar supplements).

Below are the major benefits of L-Citrulline

1. **L-Citrulline Improves The Physical Performance:** According to research, supplementation with L-citrulline is a great way to improve both the resistance and endurance. A solid proof for that is one study, where men doing resistance training were supplemented with 8 grams of L-citrulline before their chest workouts. The effects were miraculous - the number of reps they could do after the supplementation with L-citrulline went over 52%. In addition to that, the molecule significantly decreased the muscle soreness after the training. There are many other studies on L-citrulline and its amazing effects on physical performance. Generally, about 6 grams of L-citrulline per day is enough to increase the cellular energy production during exercise by 34% for average men and women, which is a significant number having in mind the average physical capacity.

2. **L-Citrulline Helps With Erectile Dysfunction:** The ability to influence blood flow makes L-citrulline a direct advantage when it comes to erection. It is proven to give men harder erection and as such prevent erectile dysfunction. Knowing that the arteries and capillary are everywhere throughout the body, L-citrulline plays a crucial role in stimulating each of

them to work to their fullest potential. L-citrulline improves erectile dysfunction (ED) and increases the hardness of erections. Some men reported having more sex after treatment and being more satisfied. Most importantly, L-citrulline prevents erectile dysfunction which is a common disorder nowadays, and it does that with zero side effects.

3. **L-Citrulline Reduces Free Radicals:** In case you don't know, free radicals are atoms or groups of atoms that can potentially cause damage to the cells in the body. While they are amazingly beneficial in many physiological processes necessary for optimal life, an excessive amount of free radicals leads to faster aging and age-dependent diseases including Cardiovascular diseases, Cancers, Neurodegenerative disorders, etc. L-citrulline steps into action by producing free radicals in the right dosage needed. While it is actively involved in the production of free radicals, it also helps the body deal with their excessive amount and reduces them accordingly.

4. **L-Citrulline Improves Heart Health:** L-citrulline is an amino acid produced naturally by the body and also found in some foods, such as watermelon, and to a lesser degree in cucumbers and cantaloupe. The body transforms L-citrulline into another amino acid, L-arginine, and also to nitric oxide. People take supplements of citrulline for erectile dysfunction and heart health as well as fatigue, dementia, muscle weakness, sickle cell disease, high blood pressure, and diabetes.

5. **L-Citrulline Helps Treat Urea Cycle Disorders:** Urea cycle disorders are genetic disorders that impair the elimination of ammonia from the body. L-Citrulline supplements can help

treat urea cycle disorders by removing ammonia from the bloodstream and preventing a build-up of it.

6. **L-Citrulline Improves Heart Function:** A study of 30 patients with heart failure found that l-citrulline increased the volume of blood pumped out of the right ventricle of the heart and lowered blood pressure in the pulmonary artery. A study of 35 patients also revealed that L-citrulline improved the function of both the right and left ventricles as well as endothelial function.

What Is The Science Behind L-Citrulline?

L-Citrulline is a naturally occurring non-essential amino acid, present in mammals and also in every living organism. It is produced by the body naturally and found naturally in certain foods such as watermelons, cucumbers, pumpkins, muskmelons, bitter melons, squashes, and gourds. About 80% of L-Citrulline (Cit) is converted in the kidney to arginine (Arg), finally converting/recycling Arg to Cit and NO and serving as a potent Arg precursor. Citrulline supplements are better for therapeutic purposes than Arg, as data show Cit supplementation elevates plasma Arg concentration and augments NO signaling in a dose-dependent manner.

Citrulline has been shown to be an effective substitute to restore nitric oxide production in situations of limited Arg availability, and Cit supplementation holds promise as a therapeutic adjunct in clinical conditions associated with Arg/NO deficiency and endothelial dysfunction.

L-citrulline is a naturally occurring amino acid found in food, such as watermelons, and also made in the body. Our bodies change L-citrulline into another amino acid called L-arginine and also to nitric oxide. L-citrulline might help increase the supply of ingredients the body needs to making certain proteins. It might also help open up veins and arteries to improve blood flow and reduce blood pressure.

L-citrulline boosts nitric oxide production in the body. Nitric oxide helps your arteries relax and work better, which improves blood flow throughout your body. This may be helpful for treating or preventing many diseases.

Evidence suggests the supplement could possibly help lower blood pressure in people with prehypertension. This is an early warning sign for high blood pressure. It means you have a slightly raised blood pressure reading of 120/80 to 139/89. Prehypertension raises your risk for high blood pressure and heart disease.

According to many studies and a lot of research, L-citrulline is a supplement that can lower the blood pressure in people who suffer from prehypertension - or act as the early warning sign for high blood pressure. This means that in a way, L-citrulline prevents high blood pressure and heart disease.

In other studies, it is shown that L-citrulline, when given to children through the vein, is a great way to prevent blood pressure complications after a heart surgery. Since it relaxes the arteries, it is helpful in this manner and ensures a proper blood flow.

L-citrulline is also linked to the prevention of erectile dysfunction; however, it does not work as well as Viagra or ED drugs used exclusively for this. Still, it is a safe option to unclog the blood vessels and stabilize the blood pressure.

How Can L-Citrulline Help Someone With Neuropathy?

Peripheral neuropathy is nerve conduction disruption that occurs outside of the central nervous system. Peripheral neuropathy (PN) can be a debilitating condition, and the cause is not always understood. Presenting symptoms often are sensory derangements, including numbness (paresthesia), hypersensitivity to mild painful stimuli (hyperesthesia), pain on light touch (allodynia), electric shock sensations (dysesthesias), and spontaneous pain without the stimulus. In more severe peripheral neuropathy, motor function impairments may present with lack of coordination, weakness, or paralysis. The autonomic nervous system may also be involved in peripheral neuropathies, and when affected, the end-organ function can be impaired. It usually presents with sensory derangements, the most debilitating of which is the pain in the extremities.

The treatment of neuropathy presents a challenge to the clinician. Opioids, anticonvulsants, antidepressants, nonsteroidal anti-inflammatory drugs, and topical agents have been used with only limited success in mitigating symptoms. Conventional therapies have limited success in preventing or reversing symptoms of neuropathic pain and numbness. In the past decade, there has been a surge in publications suggesting L-carnitine may be an effective neuroprotectant and antinociceptive for peripheral neuropathy.

L-carnitine a naturally occurring amino acid may be an ideal therapeutic agent to address this otherwise recalcitrant condition. L-Cit is potentially effective at preventing peripheral neuropathy as well as lessening neuropathic symptoms once they have developed. Both animal and human data consistently demonstrate the neuroprotective and antinociceptive effects of L-Cit. In addition, Acetyl-L-carnitine (ALC) is well tolerated without significant risk of side effects or drug-nutrient interactions. Acetyl-L-carnitine (ALC) is the ester acetylated form of carnitine, a well-characterized amino acid involved in fatty acid beta-oxidation in mitochondria.

What Exactly Does L-Citrulline Do With Blood Flow?

Citrulline produces several important effects on the body. One major way it works is by increasing vasodilation. Vasodilation refers to the widening of arteries or veins. It's associated with lower blood pressure and increased blood flow. After citrulline is consumed, some are converted to another amino acid called arginine. Arginine is converted into a molecule called nitric oxide, which causes vasodilation of blood vessels by relaxing the smooth muscle cells that constrict them.

Interestingly, consuming citrulline may increase arginine in the body more than consuming arginine itself. This is because of differences in how the body processes and absorbs arginine and citrulline. The increase in nitric oxide and blood flow may be one of the processes involved in citrulline's beneficial effects on exercise performance.

They are blood vessels that flow the blood from the heart to all of the tiny capillaries everywhere throughout the body, making sure that the body works with all of its functions. They are the link to every organ, streaming oxygenated blood directly from the heart.

Improving the ability of the blood vessels to widen can potentially improve blood pressure and blood flow to tissues. Studies have shown that a single dose of L-citrulline does not improve the ability of the arteries to widen in either healthy or diseased individuals.

However, when people who have heart disease or are at risk of heart disease have consumed L-citrulline for seven days or longer, the ability of their arteries to widen has improved. So, although a single dose may not be very effective at widening your blood vessels, taking supplements in the longer term may be more effective.

Although citrulline isn't an amino acid used directly to build proteins, it has been shown to increase protein synthesis by stimulating an important signaling pathway involved in muscle building. Citrulline may also reduce the liver's uptake of certain amino acids and prevent their breakdown.

Through these dual effects on protein synthesis and amino acid breakdown, it may contribute to maintaining or increasing muscle mass.

How Long Does It Take To See Results With L-Citrulline?

Figuring out how much you should take of a supplement can be a chore in and of itself. You certainly do not want to take too much as overdosing on anything, even supplements that are good for you can have adverse side effects. On the other hand, not getting enough will simply mean that you either won't experience any benefits, or benefits that are greatly mitigated compared to what you otherwise could get. Underdosing is actually a very common thing when supplementing with everything ranging from multivitamins to pre-workouts.

The common effective doses in the workout performance studies are between 5 and 8 grams per day. If you want to improve your exercise performance, you should take 3 to 5 grams of L-citrulline per day or 6 to 8 grams of citrulline malate per day accordingly.

Optimally, you should ingest citrulline about 15-30 minutes before training - but also during or after training if desired. If the dosage per day is too much for you to take in one go, you can increase it to 15-

20g split into multiple doses throughout the day. However, make sure to consult with your doctor before doing that.

Also, if you don't know what to expect while supplementing yourself with L-citrulline, relax. You are not the only one. In the sea of people who are easily getting excited about this supplement, it is important to note that patience is vital. After all, supplements don't build great muscles and healthy bodies - as much as your dedication to proper training and a balanced diet.

That being said, the most common results from L-citrulline as a supplement that one should expect include improved circulation, endurance, capacity, and higher energy - as well as decreased muscle soreness. In order to help you experience those results - but not overdo your supplementation - it is also important to talk about the side effects of L-citrulline.

While L-citrulline has been shown to be extremely safe when used appropriately, possible side effects, while mild, have included upset stomach. Also, some research has noted that L-citrulline can interact negatively with certain medications so be sure to consult a qualified healthcare professional before supplementing with it.

What Does L-Citrulline Do To The Cardiovascular System?

The cardiovascular system consists of the heart, blood vessels, and the approximately 5 liters of blood that the blood vessels transport. Responsible for transporting oxygen, nutrients, hormones, and cellular waste products throughout the body, the cardiovascular system is powered by the body's hardest-working organ — the heart, which is only about the size of a closed fist. The primary function of the heart and blood vessels is to transport oxygen, nutrients, and byproducts of metabolism.

L-citrulline is the natural precursor of L-arginine, a substrate for nitric oxide synthase (NOS) in the production of NO. Supplemental administration L-arginine has been shown to be effective in improving NO production and cardiovascular function in cardiovascular diseases associated with endothelial dysfunction, such as hypertension, heart failure, atherosclerosis, diabetic vascular disease, and ischemia-reperfusion injury, but the beneficial actions do not endure with chronic therapy.

L-citrulline entering the kidney, vascular endothelium and other tissues can be readily converted to L-arginine, thus raising plasma and tissue levels of L-arginine and enhancing NO production. Therefore, improving blood circulation allows more for oxygen and nutrients to flow throughout the body. Blood circulation is an important marker for cardiovascular health and influences exercise performance.

In addition to boosting exercise capacity, citrulline has also been demonstrated to improve exercise performance for both cardiovascular exercise and weight training, as well as for both aerobic (low intensity) and anaerobic (high intensity) activity. Citrulline has also been shown to be effective in reducing muscle fatigue after exercise, helping to promote recovery.

Research has shown that both L-citrulline and citrulline malate provide significant boosts to both exercise performance and cardiovascular health when taken in sufficient doses. Citrulline is very well absorbed in the body and provides numerous benefits in terms of both health and exercise performance. The benefits include: improving blood circulation, decreasing blood pressure and its associated complications, improving exercise performance, boosting immunity, promoting healing and muscle recovery after exercise by reducing muscle soreness and helping to reduce fatigue.

What Does L-Citrulline Do To The Blood Flow?

These are just some of the reasons why people turn to ingredients like L-citrulline but are these claims validated by science? What you commonly hear is that citrulline boosts nitric oxide and that's why it gives better workouts, but as we'll see, that's not entirely the case. This amino acid has also competed with ingredients like L-arginine and nitrates for boosting blood flow and catching a pump during a workout as many companies have switched back and forth between them or have outright gone back to arginine despite the research showing that citrulline is superior.

Let's first talk about citrulline in general. It is an amino acid that is involved in the urea and nitric oxide cycles and via several enzyme steps, will be converted into argininosuccinate, then into arginine, then to ornithine and back into citrulline. It works similarly in the nitric oxide cycle minus the ornithine step but plays a key role in the body's endogenous production of nitric oxide, a signaling molecule that is primarily used to relax smooth muscle in the arteries and lead to better blood flow.

Citrulline actually can raise nitric oxide production more than arginine, and can actually increase blood levels of all of the amino acids involved in the nitric oxide cycle more than arginine. It actually raises blood levels of arginine more than arginine supplementation itself! If you're stuck on the marketing surrounding arginine as a nitric oxide supplement, then you're probably better off switching to citrulline.

As far as the effects of citrulline on blood flow and blood pressure, several studies have demonstrated a slight reduction in blood pressure with supplementation. The decrease in blood pressure isn't very remarkable and appears to only occur in those with hypertension or otherwise impaired blood flow.

Now, nitric oxide itself has interesting effects on blood flow, where it relaxes the smooth muscles in the arteries and leads to an improved ability of blood to circulate. Nitric oxide production is also ramped up with dietary nitrites and nitrates and in response to increases in blood pressure.

Chapter 17

HOW THE REBUILDER SYSTEM CAN IMPROVE YOUR NEUROPATHY

T he Rebuilder is a noninvasive hand-held device approved by the FDA for the treatment of pain. This treatment device was designed based on the premise that oxygen deficiency is responsible for physical atrophy of nerve cells, which leads to the enlargement of the synaptic junction between the axon of one cell and the dendrites of the next. As a result, it is more difficult for normal-intensity electrical impulses to jump across this synaptic gap, ultimately causing neuropathy. The Rebuilder is designed to circumvent this gap by waking up dormant nerve cells, relaxing shrinking nerve cells, and restoring normal plus/minus polarity along the nerve axons and dendrites. The Rebuilder is effective for hands, knees, elbows, back, feet, and legs.

It is a specialized unit that can produce a dramatic improvement in the reduction of painful symptoms. It is an electronic device used in the privacy of your own home and is fully registered by the FDA. It is extremely dangerous to use traditional TENS or EMS device to treat neuropathy as it can overload the nerves causing permanent damage. The Rebuilder sends a very specific signal to your feet, hands, and legs that travel up and down and is an exact duplicate of a normal nerve signal.

Think of it like this-When you were young, you probably sat with your leg under your buttocks and your leg "fell asleep." Your leg tingled, and you began to feel numbness. So what did Mother Nature have you do? You simply moved your leg (stopping the cause) and stomped your foot on the ground, and the feeling in your leg returned. This worked because you sent a much larger, but normal nerve impulse up your leg to the nerve roots of your lower back. That is exactly how the Rebuilder works!

What Is It Used For?

The Rebuilder is a small, hand-held, battery-powered nerve stimulator that sends a comfortable electronic impulse to your feet and legs. It is a patient-friendly device that can be used to treat neuropathic pain. It requires a 30-minute treatment window in which the patient applies conductive gel to each of the signal pads. The pads are then placed on the soles of the feet, the palms of the hands, the lower back, or the shoulders, as needed.

It also knows what area of the body you are using the unit on due to the different waveforms that are being sensed by the machine. This is a unique safety feature of the Rebuilder; no other unit offers this level of safety.

The Rebuilder accomplishes various functions in a simple to use home care system that is not only effective in helping relieve many of the symptoms of neuropathy and chronic pain and in limiting its progression but can cause the regression of pain, burning, and numbness. When the Rebuilder's electrical signals stimulate the leg muscles to contract, this "venous muscle pump" moves the mineral-rich blood to the muscles and the nerves. Osmotic pressure and the ionic tension from the Rebuilder's signals successfully jumping across the gaps then carries these necessary minerals into the synaptic junctions between the nerve cells helping to restore the conductivity that is characteristically lost.

As part of its uses, the Rebuilder system contributes to the healing process by accomplishing the following:

- Stimulates leg muscles to contract and relax thereby increasing blood velocity and volume with fresh blood to the nerves and muscles.
- Stimulates all the afferent and efferent nerves in the lower extremities with a signal larger than normal to re-establish the pathways for subsequent normal signals to follow.
- Draws axon and dendrite nerve endings closer together to facilitate proper nerve transmission.
- Causes the brain to release endorphins that reduce global pain and anxiety.
- Promotes the healing of non-plantar surface diabetic skin ulcers and sprains.
- Increases muscle strength for safe, pain-free walking.
- Reduces edema as muscle contractions encourage lymphatic drainage and movement to the proper nodes.

How does The Rebuilder System Work?

The Rebuilder work by sending its healing signals to your feet, hands or back. Small conductive rubber signal pads are placed on your skin. Then, you simply sit back and relax for your treatment. This excellent device uses a tiny electrical signal to wake up nerves that are temporarily dormant or asleep. These signals mimic your natural nerve signals but are stronger. This signal travels from one foot, up the leg, across the synaptic junctions and nerve roots in your lower back and down to the other foot. Then it reverses polarity and travels back to the original foot. This back and forth action effectively treats all the nerves of both legs and feet.

At the same time, your calf muscles and contracting and relaxing, as they would naturally during exercise like walking. An additional benefit results from the brain releasing endorphins, strong pain relievers that travel in the bloodstream to all parts of the body. These natural pain relievers are known to relieve depression and physical pain without any adverse side effects. The Rebuilder opens up the nerve paths, re-educating them to transmit normal nerve signals to the brain. The resulting increased blood flow results in a therapeutic healing process, not a temporary fix.

Imagine no side effects, walking pain-free, no fear of stumbling, sleeping through the night and feeling the carpet and grass under your feet! The ReBuilder can give you these results along with the benefits of reducing or stopping the need for drugs and pain medications, relieving your pain and numbness and restoring your mobility.

How Does The Rebuilder System Compare To A Traditional TENS Unit?

The Rebuilder System is totally different from any other treatment system offered anywhere in the world to treat the painful symptoms of nerve pain (neuropathy). The Rebuilder's built-in microprocessor measures several physiological functions of your nerves and automatically adjusts itself to your specific therapeutic needs beginning with the first healing signal. While sitting in your chair or bed, this signal travels automatically from one foot, up the leg, across the nerve roots in the lower back, then down the other leg to the other foot.

The Rebuilder's Impulses utilize very small amounts of current under the curve and a relatively high transient voltage of 40-90 volts. The resultant current is below that commonly produced by traditional TENS units. The device delivers a second, simultaneous, lower voltage (5-20 volts), wider waveform signal designed to stimulate muscle tissue. This signal causes the muscles of the feet, calves, and thighs and buttocks to intermittently contract and relax. Stimulating the venous muscle pump to empty veins thus allowing whatever arterial pressure is present to fill the vacated veins rapidly. This enhances local blood flow.

Also, the Rebuilder utilizes multiple bio-feedback loops that enable the device to measure and analyze the patient's nerve function before, during, and after the treatment. This means that every 12 hundredths of a second the Rebuilder is responding to your individual physiological status, creating, and delivering a unique signal.

As for other traditional TENS unit, It is extremely dangerous to use a common TENS or EMS device to treat neuropathy as it can overload the nerves causing permanent damage. The Rebuilder sends a very specific signal to your feet, hands, and legs that travel up and down and is an exact duplicate of a normal nerve signal. Rather than simply numbing your nerves like drugs or other TENS-like devices (essentially ineffective and potentially dangerous "toys"), the Rebuilder can calm down your overactive nerves and wake up your under-active nerves. Also, the Rebuilder's healing signals include electronic muscle stimulation which automatically strengthens nearby calf muscles (or arm muscles when used for hand pain), and increases local blood flow to enhance permanent healing.

What Are The Different Types Of Neuropathy's That The Rebuilder System Can Help With?

Neuropathy is defined as a disease (pathos) of the nerves (neuro). It is the damage to the nerves of the peripheral nervous system, which may be caused either by disease of or trauma to the nerve or the side effects of systemic illness. Simply put at some time in the past, your nerves were challenged and to protect themselves from the additional damage they became dormant.

In fact, neuropathy, which is sometimes referred to as peripheral neuropathy, is not a single health condition but rather a term used to describe a range of health problems involving damage to the peripheral nerves, as well as the symptoms of those issues.

There are four types of diabetic neuropathy:

Peripheral Neuropathy: Peripheral diabetic neuropathy goes by various names: peripheral diabetic nerve pain and distal polyneuropathy. Peripheral neuropathy is the most common form of neuropathy caused by diabetes. It affects nerves leading to your extremities to your feet, legs, hands, and arms. The nerves going to your feet are the longest in your body: after they branch off the spinal cord in the lumbar region (low back), they have to go all the way down your legs and into the feet quite a distance. Because the nerves leading to your feet are so long, it's most often these nerves that are damaged; there are more of them to be damaged. This nerve damage can lead to the foot problems often associated with diabetes, including foot deformities, infections, ulcers, and amputations.

Proximal Neuropathy: Proximal neuropathy can also be called diabetic amyotrophy. That myo in the word means muscle, so this is a form of neuropathy that can cause muscle weakness. It specifically affects the muscles in the upper part of your leg(s), buttocks, and hips. Proximal neuropathy is the second most common type of diabetic neuropathy (second only to peripheral diabetic neuropathy). It usually affects older adults with diabetes; as opposed to peripheral neuropathy, it usually resolves with time or treatment.

Autonomic Neuropathy: Autonomic nerves are supposed to keep your body running as it should. There are many functions that happen in your body without you thinking about them: your heart pumps, you breathe, and your stomach digests food. The autonomic nervous system controls those actions; it's also sometimes called the automatic nervous system. The autonomic nervous system should maintain your body's homeostasis, which is its normal, balanced state. Autonomic neuropathy can seem daunting because it can affect so many of your body's systems, from your digestive tract to how well you can see. However, remember that your symptoms depend on what specific nerves in the autonomic nervous system are damaged.

Focal Neuropathy: All of the types of diabetic neuropathy above— peripheral, autonomic, and proximal—are examples of polyneuropathy. Poly means that they affect many nerves. Focal neuropathy, by contrast, affects one specific nerve; it's focused neuropathy. It can also be called mononeuropathy. Focal neuropathy, which comes on suddenly, most often affects nerves in the head (especially ones that go to the eyes). It can also affect the torso and legs.

When focal neuropathy affects the legs, it has different symptoms than proximal neuropathy, which can also affect the legs. Proximal neuropathy, as you can read above, causes muscle weakness in the legs, and it may also cause shooting pain down the leg.

What Kind Of Results Does The Rebuilder System Produce?

The Rebuilder is a noninvasive hand-held device approved by the FDA for the treatment of pain. This treatment device was designed based on the premise that oxygen deficiency is responsible for physical atrophy of nerve cells, which leads to the enlargement of the synaptic junction between the axon of one cell and the dendrites of the next. As a result, it is more difficult for normal-intensity electrical impulses to jump across this synaptic gap, ultimately causing neuropathy. The Rebuilder is designed to circumvent this gap by waking up dormant nerve cells, relaxing shrinking nerve cells, and restoring normal plus/minus polarity along the nerve axons and dendrites.

The Rebuilder works simultaneously on three separate levels: stimulation of the nerves, stimulation of the muscles, and combined electrostimulation.

The first signal is designed to stimulate the nerves by sending an electrical impulse with a very narrow wave-form and a relatively high transient voltage: 40 to 90 volts AC. The resulting current is miniscule and much below what is commonly found with traditional TENS devices. A larger than normal signal must be used because of the widening gap between the nerve cells and the loss of much of the conductivity in the synaptic junction fluid due to demineralization the Rebuilder's nerve stimulation signal is many times stronger than the normal afferent and efferent signals; therefore, it can effectively complete the circuit. This stimulates the nerves causing them to re-establish their normal metabolic function. This signal, crossing the synaptic junctions, also re-polarizes the junctions causing them to be receptive to reabsorb minerals thus improving the conductivity.

The second signal stimulates the muscles by a different, wider waveform with a larger subthreshold amount of current under the curve and a much smaller voltage (5 to 20 AC). Muscles are most responsive to this waveform. This signal causes the muscles of the feet, calves, thighs, and buttocks to contract and relax in harmony with the Rebuilder's signal. Overcoming any residual inflammatory resistance to blood flow, the Rebuilder's proprietary signal also has specific characteristics that cause a complete relaxation of the muscles' fast and slow twitch cells between each contraction stimulus.

The third signal is the combined electrostimulation. This twin electrical signal (one to stimulate the nerve cells and the other to trigger muscle cells) is pulsed on and off at the frequency of 7.83 cycles per second. One postulation for this sensitivity is that the electrical potential between the earth's atmosphere and the earth's surface is also approximately 7.83 Hz. Simultaneously stimulating the muscles of the feet, calves, thighs, and buttocks, the Rebuilder evokes complete relaxation between each contraction stimulus. This increases the flow of oxygen-rich blood to the synaptic junctions, affording effective and efficient conduction of nerve signals. Combined electro¬

stimulation uses twin electrical signals to stimulate the nerves and muscle cells.

Using this signal frequency, the body not only responds favorably but the brain is induced to release large amounts of endorphins. The manufacturer states that the twin electrical signals cause the brain to release endorphins, producing a sense of well-being and reducing anxiety as well as physical and emotional trauma. Endorphins, internal analgesics as powerful as and chemically related to morphine but without any negative side effects, are created and modulated by the body's chemistry. The impact of this endorphin release is a generalized sense of well-being, a reduction in pain and anxiety levels elsewhere in the body, and even a reduction in emotional pain. Reduction of pain will lead to improvement in patient compliance and quality of life.

Additionally, the Rebuilder features a simultaneous weighted DC signal designed to stabilize the trigger threshold that regulates the sensitivity of the nerve cell. By sending this constant DC signal, the resting potential is held at a fixed voltage long enough for the cell to stabilize itself and regain control.

What Are The Contraindications Associated With The Rebuilder System?

There are no negative side effects when using the Rebuilder system according to the directions. However, we have had reports of sore or cramping calf muscles resulting from using it at too high a setting for a sustained period, much like exercising too much too quickly. It is recommended that you use the Rebuilder initially at a low setting thereby allowing the feet and legs time to adjust to the stimulation. On a rare occasion, an individual may experience a headache or nausea. This infrequent reaction can happen as a result of an adrenalin rush for users who harbor a latent fear of electricity as a whole. That subconscious fear can produce adrenalin that, in turn, produces temporary headaches or nausea. There are, however, positive side effects of using the unit. As a result of nerve stimulation, the brain releases endorphins which help relax muscles and reduce pain in other parts of the body. The Rebuilder system also helps to increase mobility by building muscle mass, improving leg strength, and promoting better balance. In addition, many clients also report experiencing a better night rest and a reduction in the need for pain medication.

How Long Does It Take To Begin To See Benefits With The Rebuilder System?

As with any treatment, results vary from individual to individual. Some clients report immediate results and, again, there are some who reported positive results after as much as five to seven months. Response to treatment is governed by many factors, such as whether or not the individual is dealing with multiple medical conditions in addition to numbers of and classes of prescription drugs they may be taking. It has been our experience, however, that individuals who are persistent in following their treatment regimen will ultimately gain an improvement in their condition.

Finally, the Rebuilder treatment for nerve pain (neuropathy) is safe, effective, without side effects, and very easy to use. You will experience immediate, total relief from your symptoms during your first 30-min treatment at home. After your 30 minute treatment, you will experience a 50%-70% reduction in your symptoms for 3-4 hours. When used before bedtime you will fall asleep faster and sleep comfortably throughout the night.

Chapter 18

THE FUTURE OF HEALING
HAS ARRIVED

The healthcare world is full of treatment options based on medications, surgery, and preventive and palliative care; however, the new world has newer options for improved treatment technologies. Technology based on quantum mechanics has a different way of looking at our medical health issues. It has simple principles that can alter the basis of medical techniques and even our own biology. It uses the resonance energy between the cells and tissues that help provide adequate energy to the target body site to reach the intended goal. The principle can be understood from the resonance energy emitted from the tuning forks that strikes that piano tuner. When the frequency of both the tuners match, the vibration produced makes the intended piano sound.

Sanexas System

Sanexas System works on the basis of Electrical Cell Signaling (ECsT). The mechanism of the Sanexas system is based on successive depolarization and repolarization of the muscles. There are two types of classes that belong to this system, i.e., the stimulating System, which involves consecutive polarization and repolarization to inflict excitatory potential, and the multi-facilitation class, which involves no action potential but only some effects of biochemical nature. The stimulatory class is used for treating analgesia, resolving circulatory and lymphatic issues, reducing edema, and accelerating regeneration processes in the body. The multi-facilitation class is more suitable for anti-inflammatory actions and edema management, along with the other issues included in the stimulatory class therapy choices.

Discovery of Senaxes System

The concept of pain treatment is based on the Quantum Resonance-Specific Induction QRSI. The model proposes the idea of impacting electromagnetic energy in the form of electric currents in the bone and joint area. This will generate electrical impulses in the affected area and result in the amplification of resonating subatomic particles in the cells and tissues. This resonating energy is responsible for pain amelioration and healing. This technique works by increasing the cellular electron transport across cell membranes to enhance polarity. This also increases microtubular conduction within the cell and induces capacitance in the cell membranes. The method improves cellular energy and communication within the cells and also improves the functions of organs and tissues.

Principle and Mechanism of Senaxes System

All the new technologies based on quantum mechanics follow the principle of Electrical Cell Signaling (ECsT), but there are some special features in the Senaxes System that make it different from all others.

All of these operate using amplitude modulated (AM) electrotechnical devices and generate multi-facilitated frequencies. The Senaxes System makes use of both the frequency-modulated (FM) and amplitude modulated (AM) signals, as well as a unique System called frequency-hopping spread spectrum (FHSS) that has the potential to deliver both low frequency and middle-frequency signals. The simultaneous delivery of AM and FM generates electrical impulses along the axon line, very much like the physiological phenomenon making the therapeutic effect possible. The mechanism by which the pain relief is experienced through Senaxes System includes the pH variation, enhanced trophic movements, better intercellular communication, imitated movements of neuronal hormones and ligands, augmented cAMP activation, and better permeability of the cell membranes.

Applications of Sanexas System - The Real Expectations

It is definitely a greater preference over the Transcutaneous Electrical Nerve Stimulation therapy because it offers a Systematic relief from acute, chronic pain, and post-traumatic pain. It can also be used to treat pain after surgical procedures. Because the electrical impulses work on the basis of vibrations, it is useful for muscular spasms as well as muscular atrophy. Immediate phlebothrombosis is another condition treatable through this method because it improves blood circulation in the body by stimulating vascular flow. People who have limited movement of a certain part of the body can be improved through the use of the Sanexas System.

Using Senaxes For Neuropathy

The frequencies, when inflicted on the targeted site of the body, which is the feet here, stay there for a limited period of time, causing vibrations in the cells and tissues of the knee. Harmonic resonance effects are imposed on the cell membranes and voltage-gated ion channels of the neurons lining the knee. These frequencies allow the cells in the knee to absorb energy which gives the power to the injury and pain to heal and recover. Electronic Signal Technology is specifically different in this aspect because it gives energy to the cells for repairing processes by inducing electromagnetic potentials at the microtubular level in the cells.

People who suffer from neuropathy can use this technology with anticipated positive results. Research shows a reduction in the use of opioids by 67% for inflammation, and injury. Interestingly, this level of improvement in neuropathy is reported within a period of 60 days of Senaxes System mediated therapy.

Calmare - Another Pain Therapy Technology

Calmare itself means to soothe or calm - hence the term directs toward the treatment of pain. It is a US Food and Drug Authority authorized technology for pain treatment. This technology was approved by the European CE as well, which makes it very popular among the latest pain treatment options. It is another non-invasive technology that allows patients suffering from consistent pain to get a sigh of relief after all. Patients undergoing treatment through Calmare would be able to surpass all the negative adverse effects like drug-associated nausea and other symptoms, addiction, behavioral dependence, and other potentially harmful and fatal effects.

Calmare device has been shown to improve skeletal as well as neuropathic pains in more than 4000 cases and is continued to be utilized in the world of pain therapy. The conditions being treated are not only limited to neck, lower back, post-injury, and post-surgery pains but also extend to the treatment of Phantom limbs syndrome, chemotherapy-associated pain, dystrophy pains, and postherpetic neuralgia.

How the Calmare system works

There is a multiprocessor installed in the device that works on biophysical methods rather than any biochemical concept. There are electrodes placed on the skin surface level on the patient's affected part of the body. The electrode catches the radio signals emitting in and out of the body that shows the pain and the no-pain areas in the body. The pain signal in the body is dominantly felt by the body and is also detected by the device as the bigger signal, making it easier to treat the pain.

There are patients that have varied intensity of pain and have for long considered alternative therapies for pain treatment. Unfortunately, declining results have left the patients with no hope making them a little less hopeful with this latest technology as well. However, this technique has modified the pain treatment success rate by curing hundreds and thousands of patients of pain. The maximum effect of the treatment can be achieved by regularly scheduling follow-up calls with the doctor. People who are absent for subsequent follow-up schedules show little to less treatment effectiveness as compared to those who show better compliance with the scheduled therapy.

The Role of Calmare In Treating Neuropathy

Calmare is a biophysical technology that is not only reserved for conditions like neuropathy but is useful for multifarious muscular and pain problems in the body. People who have had persistent untreated pain over the years are recommended to try this technology and say goodbye to the bodily pains once and for all. Patients who come up for this treatment are usually treated with an 80% reduction in the intensity of the pain. Calmare has been evidently known for treating neuropathic pains as well as Failed Back Surgery Syndrome, sciatic and lumbar pains, post-surgical and post-injury pains, as well as Phantom Limb Syndrome.

Neurogenx as the New Pain Relieving System

Neurogenx is the latest technology being used for the treatment of chronic and never-ending pain conditions. It is a non-invasive and non-narcotic technique which means that people who have been suffering from the side effects of drug dependence and surgical complications can now skip the aggressive steps and jump directly to easier nervous stimulations for pain relief. This electro-medical technique has increased the number of successful cases quite speedily all across the states of America. The technology makes use of high frequency, cutting edge technology, the rays of which penetrate deep down into the muscular tissues and joints, making the therapy more efficient and substantial than before.

The treatment by Neurogenx works at a cellular level, thereby reducing swelling and inflammation from the point of origin in the tissues. It increases the metabolism and enhances the excretion of waste products so that the cells can repair themselves with their maximum rapid potential. So far, the traditional options for treating neuropathy involve long-term follow-ups and frequent therapy segments, which still lead to incompetent and unsatisfactory results. Neurogenx has upgraded the level of expectation a patient keeps from the possible cure rate provided and is a knockout for all the current pain therapy options available.

The Principles of The Neurogenx Pain Treatment

Neurogenx provides patients the hope of maximum to complete pain relief. The patients enrolled in the clinical trials have shown as much as an 87% success rate. The Neurogenx device contains certain electrodes constituting patches that are adhesive in nature. These are attached to the affected part of the body, exactly where the patient complains of pain. This means that the electrodes are placed on the exact anatomical part of neuropathy by the assistant physician. The changes are then inflicted on a cellular level to increase the rate of metabolism in the cells of the affected area. This happens with the help of pH variation, bringing it back to the normal values. It also takes place by eliminating excess fluid from the affected part so that the removal of waste speeds up and healing takes place as quickly as possible.

The Use of Neurogenx with Neuropathy

Neurogenx is capable of treating neuropathic pain by the same mechanism that follows the repair and healing of other conditions. The pain can be associated with damage to the ligaments and tendons, or it can be directly linked to the deterioration in the joint, a nearby bone, or the attached muscles. Medical science is still exploring the method of cell function in neurons and how they regenerate. Although the mechanism is unknown, the process itself can be used to interfere with the natural phenomenon and augment it to accelerate cellular repair.

The knee conditions will be treated by Neurogenx by the advanced medical protocols that will not only treat the pains of varying intensities but will also re-establish pain sensation and other neural sensations, making the normal movement of the knee joint[9] possible once again.

Neuropathic Conditions Treated by Neurogenx

The treatment for neuropathy related conditions under the Neurogenx therapy usually involves a series of therapies and spans a period of 4 to 6 weeks. Although the number of sessions might seem long, improvement is usually noticed by patients within the first 2 to 3 sessions which is faster compared to any other alternative therapy available. People who have fibromyalgia are usually not able to walk or even bend their knees. Chemotherapeutic patients[10] feel numbness and needle-like pricking in the knees and the legs. There are people injured because of severe physical trauma, having damaged cartilage and deteriorated synovial membranes in case of arthritis. All of these conditions are treatable through Neurogenx Pain Therapy.

Extracorporeal Magnetotransduction Therapy (EMTT)

Extraxcorporeal Magnetotransduction Therapy or EMTT is another non-invasive form of treatment that is now increasingly being used to treat musculoskeletal pain and relieve the patients' from their chronic pain and discomfort-related symptoms. It is different from its related, non-invasive modes of treatment in a way because it employs higher oscillatory waves and much stronger electromagnetic fields when being used on the patient. It is said that it is because of these enhanced and increased electromagnetic powers that EMTT proves to be a remarkable and greatly pain-relieving modality for reliving patient's pain and discomfort within a few sessions.

The Principle Of How EMTT Works

Once the treatment begins, the painful or tender areas are kept under focus of the Electromagnetic Therapy Machine. This machine keeps on emitting magnetic pulses or waves periodically. Usually, these waves are under the range of 10 milliTesla, but the range may vary depending on the severity of the symptoms being experienced by the patient under treatment.

Once this magnetic field has established and is in 'running' position, several effects start taking place all at once in the area under focus. The membrane potential stabilizes itself and once this happens, ion channels also open up and thus, an active exchange gradient is set up. These very effects have been seen to accelerate the healing processes, which in turn help the person heal from their chronic pain conditions within a short period of undergoing these sessions.

EMTT And Its Role In Neuropathic Related Conditions

EMTT has been seen to be particularly helpful in treating neuropathy-related conditions. The reason for this is that instead of being helpful for large regions of the body, EMTT has been found to be particularly helpful in treating the smaller or localized regions of the body, since the machine can focus on such areas in a better way.

In the context of the feet, the same thing happens because the feet are held under the machine under full focus. There are several acute and chronic conditions of the knee that can be easily treated using this mode of therapy. Neuropathy related disorders and other inflammatory conditions, and several other traumatic feet related injuries have been effectively treated using this modality.

EMTT indeed is a helpful and worthy mode of treatment that can help treat small but persistent pain conditions in no time.

Made in United States
Orlando, FL
02 June 2022

18426061R00137